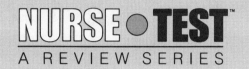

DOSAGE
CALCULATIONS

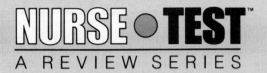

DOSAGE CALCULATIONS

June Looby Olsen, RN, MS
Professor of Nursing
College of Staten Island
Staten Island, N.Y.

Eugenia Borgia Murray, RN, BA
Manager, Nursing Skills Laboratory
Department of Nursing
College of Staten Island
Staten Island, N.Y.

Series Editor
Laura Gasparis Vonfrolio, RN, MA, CCRN, CEN
Assistant Professor of Nursing
College of Staten Island
Staten Island, N.Y.

Springhouse Corporation
Springhouse, Pennsylvania

Staff

Executive Director, Editorial
Stanley Loeb

Director of Trade and Textbooks
Minnie B. Rose, RN, BSN, MEd

Art Director
John Hubbard

Clinical Consultant
Maryann Foley, RN, BSN

Editors
Mary Durkin, Diane Labus, David Moreau

Copy Editor
Mary Hohenhaus Hardy

Designers
Stephanie Peters (associate art director), Julie Carleton Barlow

Art Production
Robert Perry (manager), Anna Brindisi, Donald Knauss, Tom Robbins, Robert Wieder

Typography
David Kosten (director), Diane Paluba (manager), Elizabeth Bergman, Joyce Rossi Biletz, Phyllis Marron, Robin Rantz, Valerie Rosenberger

Manufacturing
Deborah Meiris (manager), T.A. Landis, Jennifer Suter

Ⓡ A member of the Reed Elsevier plc group

Library of Congress Cataloging-in-Publication Data

Olsen, June Looby.
    Dosage calculations/June Looby
    Olsen, Eugenia Borgia Murray.
        p.   cm. — (NurseTest)
    Includes bibliographical references.
    1. Pharmaceutical arithmetic —
Examinations, questions, etc.   I. Murray,
Eugenia Borgia.   II. Title.   III. Series.
    [DNLM: 1. Drugs — administration &
dosage — examination questions.
2. Mathematics — examination questions.
3. Nursing Care — examination questions. WY
18 052d]
RS57.048 1992
615.5'8 — dc20
DNLM/DLC   91-4828
ISBN 0-87434-301-1   CIP

Contents

Acknowledgments and Dedications

We wish to thank those people who enabled this book to become a reality: Laura Gasparis Vonfrolio, for her encouragement, confidence in us, and remarkable ability to share; each other, for mutual respect, love, and work ethics; our families, for their unending patience; Mary Geisler, for her endurance and typing expertise; Springhouse Publishing Company, for having confidence in this project; and all our students, who have eagerly awaited publication of this book.

For all my nephews — Steven and Emil Petagna; Carl, Gary, Mike, Shawn, and Patrick Looby; Don and Chris Dingman; and, last but not least, Billie, Scot, and Marshall Looby.

J.L.O.

In loving memory of my father, James C. Borgia.

E.B.M.

Preface

This book is one in a series designed to help nursing students, professional licensed or registered nurses, nurses educated abroad, and nurses returning to the field improve their test-taking skills and increase their theoretical knowledge of nursing. It features case-study situations and a multiple-choice question-and-answer format similar to that used in NCLEX-RN (National Council Licensure Examination for Registered Nurses) and nursing challenge examinations. It also includes a comprehensive examination to test overall knowledge of questions and answers presented in each of the chapters.

Dosage Calculations offers hundreds of sample problems to test basic computation and conversion skills needed by those who prepare and administer dosages or who monitor patients receiving drugs or I.V. fluids in a clinical setting. Topics focus on:
- understanding the metric and apothecaries' systems
- converting between systems
- calculating nonparenteral and parenteral dosages
- preparing and administering I.V. solutions
- calculating and preparing pediatric dosages
- working through complex calculations.

Solutions to problems are provided using both dimensional analysis and ratio and proportion—the two most commonly used methods for determining dosage calculations. A quick-reference list of the most common abbreviations in drug therapy can be found in the Appendix.

When using this book, remember to begin with the first question in each chapter and proceed in a sequential manner. Do not skip around, since subsequent answers may build on previous ones.

Introduction

Nurses are tested continually throughout their careers — as nursing students in the classroom, as professionals undergoing licensure or certification, and as practicing clinicians in the health care delivery field. Such testing helps to measure acquired knowledge and ultimately prepares nurses for real-life clinical situations.

Because testing knowledge is an important, ongoing aspect of a nurse's career and heavy emphasis is placed upon passing certain critical examinations, such as NCLEX-RN (National Council Licensure Examination for Registered Nurses) and nursing challenge examinations, nurses must rely on practical study guides and effective test-taking strategies if they are to succeed.

NurseTest: A Review Series was developed to help nurses improve their test-taking abilities and increase their general clinical knowledge. Each book in the series focuses on a specific area of study or a speciality of nursing practice. Written in a question-and-answer format, each book includes hundreds of questions built on case-study situations and a final comprehensive examination that tests overall subject knowledge. All questions, which appear at the beginning of each chapter, include four possible answers. The correct answers — along with rationales, when applicable — appear at the end of each chapter. A blank answer sheet is provided in each chapter.

Although having a thorough understanding of the clinical material is probably the best way to ensure a good test result, developing and implementing good test-taking strategies may mean the difference between passing and failing. Such strategies include physical and mental preparation, paying attention to directions, keeping track of the time, and reading the questions and answer choices carefully to determine the most appropriate response.

Preparing for the test

Regardless of your reason for taking the test, you'll need to be prepared. If you are like many nurses, this may mean extensive reading, note taking, studying, and reviewing. Therefore, developing good study habits is vital. Whether studying alone or in a group, you'll do well to follow a few simple rules:

• Find a place that is conducive to studying, such as a library, study hall, or lounge, if distractions are a problem.

• Limit your studying to several short sessions rather than one long cramming session.

• Highlight only the most essential information, and take selective notes.

• Concentrate on the most difficult or least familiar information first, saving the most familiar information for last.

• Anticipate feeling some anxiety over the test, but try to find ways to relieve it. For example, try practicing deep-breathing exercises and other forms of relaxation, such as rhythmically tensing and relaxing muscle groups throughout your body. Practicing such exercises the night before the test and even while the papers are being distributed alleviates tension and promotes better concentration.

After what seems like countless hours of studying for an important test, the most effective final preparation is to relax and take it easy. Last-minute cramming can do little to increase knowledge and may cause unneeded stress and fatigue. Exercising or going to a movie the night before the test — then getting a good night's sleep — is usually most helpful.

Taking the test

Before answering any questions, remember to focus on the cardinal rules of test taking:

• Pay attention to directions.

• Read all instructions and questions carefully.

• Answer only what is being asked; do not read into a question anything beyond what is there.

• Know how much time is allotted for the test, and pace yourself accordingly. Be sure to note the halfway time.

• Scan the first page for a question you can answer easily, and mark the answer in the appropriate space on the answer sheet. Then go back to the first question and begin answering the questions in consecutive order. Answering an easy question first may give you a boost of confidence.

• Do not spend excessive time on any one question. If a question seems too difficult or complex, skip the question but remember to circle the number on the answer sheet; then return to the question after completing the other questions.

• Never leave an answer blank or mark two choices for the same answer.

• Compare the test to the answer sheet periodically to ensure that you haven't made any slight but costly errors, such as answering question 4 in question 5's space on the answer sheet.

• Erase all stray marks from the answer sheet before handing in the test.

Choosing the correct response

In a multiple-choice test, determining the correct answer to a question can sometimes be difficult. However, in many cases, you can successfully determine the correct answer by using one or more of the strategies listed below:

• Eliminate any obviously incorrect choices; then, reevaluate the remaining options and choose the most likely response. Ideally, you should try to narrow your choices to two likely options, affording yourself a 50% chance of choosing the correct answer. If choosing between the two remaining options seems especially difficult, take an educated guess.

• Look for key words or phrases in the question that can point to a correct response. For example, questions including the words "best," "most appropriate," or "most accurate" usually suggest that the correct response is a true statement, whereas those including "all...except," "least effective," and "least appropriate" usually suggest a false statement as the correct response. Such key words as "immediately," "promptly," and "highest priority" usually indicate that the correct response is something a nurse would normally do first.

• Look for interlocking clues, in which the correct response to one question forms the basis of the next question:

---

1 The nurse is caring for Mr. P., who is exhibiting abnormal extension and adduction of the arms, pronation of the wrists, and flexion of the fingers. Which type of posturing is characterized by such abnormalities?

A. Decorticate
B. Apraxic
C. Akinetic
D. Decerebrate

---

2 The nurse explains to Mr. P.'s daughter that decerebrate posturing typically results from:

A. Temporary lack of oxygen to the brain
B. Infection
C. Brain stem damage
D. Extrapyramidal system damage

In this example, "decerebrate" (the focus of the second question) is the correct answer to the first question. Although the mere repetition of "decerebrate" might suggest that it is the correct response, the real interlocking clue lies in the logical transition from one question to the other: in this case, the nurse cares for a patient exhibiting abnormal posturing, then explains the nature of such posturing to the patient's daughter.

Important: When looking for interlocking clues, always remember to read the questions and answer choices carefully, as choosing an answer solely on the basis of its repetition in another question can sometimes backfire:

---

1 Which type of posturing is characterized by abnormal flexion and adduction of the arms and by flexion of the fingers and wrists on the chest?

A. Decorticate
B. Apraxic
C. Akinetic
D. Decerebrate

2 The nurse understands that decerebrate posturing typically results from:

A. Temporary lack of oxygen to the brain
B. Infection
C. Brain stem damage
D. Extrapyramidal system damage

In this second example, "decerebrate" appears as an answer choice in the first question as well as the focus of the second question. Despite its repetition, however, "decerebrate" is not the correct response to the first question ("decorticate" is correct). The two questions are independent of each other, and no logical transition (or interlocking clue) exists.

After the test
Once you have completed the test, try to put it out of your mind; nothing can change the outcome at this point. Later, however, take time to review the test, if you're given an opportunity to do so — reviewing the questions and answers may provide some insight for future experiences. Otherwise, be satisfied with your accomplishment, and resume your usual work and leisure activities while you wait for the results. And expect to be pleasantly surprised.

Alice Geraghty Graham, RN, BSN, MS, MA
Assistant Professor of Nursing
College of Staten Island
Staten Island, N.Y.

CHAPTER 1

Metric System

Questions

1 0.6 g equals how many milligrams?

A. 10 mg
B. 24 mg
C. 60 mg
D. 600 mg

2 30 mg equal how many micrograms?

A. 10,000 mcg
B. 30,000 mcg
C. 90,000 mcg
D. None of the above

3 10 kg equal how many grams?

A. 100 g
B. 1,000 g
C. 10,000 g
D. 100,000 g

4 0.03 mg equals how many grams?

A. 0.000003 g
B. 0.00003 g
C. 0.0009 g
D. 0.009 g

5 0.75 g equals how many milligrams?

A. 7.5 mg
B. 75 mg
C. 750 mg
D. 7,500 mg

6 4.8 kg equal how many grams?

A. 48 g
B. 480 g
C. 4,800 g
D. 48,000 g

7 750 mg equal how many grams?

A. 0.75 g
B. 7.5 g
C. 75 g
D. 750 g

8 0.0002 g equals how many milligrams?

    A. 0.2 mg
    B. 200 mg
    C. 2,000 mg
    D. 22,000 mg

9 0.2 g equals how many milligrams?

    A. 0.0002 mg
    B. 0.04 mg
    C. 20 mg
    D. 200 mg

10 How many milligrams are in 3 g of a drug?

    A. 0.6 mg
    B. 30 mg
    C. 3,000 mg
    D. 6,000 mg

11 0.004 g equals how many milligrams?

    A. 0.4 mg
    B. 4 mg
    C. 400 mg
    D. 4,000 mg

12 0.016 mg equals how many micrograms?

    A. 2 mcg
    B. 4 mcg
    C. 16 mcg
    D. 320 mcg

13 0.0003 g equals how many milligrams?

    A. 0.009 mg
    B. 0.09 mg
    C. 0.3 mg
    D. 9 mg

14 0.002 mg equals how many micrograms?

    A. 2 mcg
    B. 4 mcg
    C. 20 mcg
    D. 40 mcg

15 6 kg equal how many grams?

A. 60 g
B. 6,000 g
C. 60,000 g
D. 360,000 g

16 250 mcg equal how many milligrams?

A. 0.0025 mg
B. 0.005 mg
C. 0.05 mg
D. 0.25 mg

17 2.5 U equal how many milliunits?

A. 0.25 mU
B. 0.5 mU
C. 50 mU
D. 2,500 mU

18 0.25 liter equals how many milliliters?

A. 250 ml
B. 2,500 ml
C. 4,800 ml
D. 50,000 ml

19 300 mU equal how many units?

A. 0.003 U
B. 0.3 U
C. 3 U
D. 6 U

20 0.00065 g equals how many milligrams?

A. 0.00065 mg
B. 0.0143 mg
C. 0.143 mg
D. 0.65 mg

21 1 mcg equals how many milligrams?

A. 0.000001 mg
B. 0.00001 mg
C. 0.001 mg
D. 1,000 mg

22 600 mg equal how many grams?

    A. 0.06 g
    B. 0.6 g
    C. 6 g
    D. 60 g

23 0.25 mg equals how many micrograms?

    A. 0.025 mcg
    B. 25 mcg
    C. 250 mcg
    D. 500 mcg

24 A patient is to receive 300 mg of a drug that is available only in grams. How many grams should the nurse administer?

    A. 0.0003 g
    B. 0.006 g
    C. 0.06 g
    D. 0.3 g

25 If a patient is to be given 10 mg of a drug, what would be the equivalent dose in grams?

    A. 0.01 g
    B. 1 g
    C. 100 g
    D. 1,000 g

Answer sheet

	A	B	C	D
1	○	○	○	○
2	○	○	○	○
3	○	○	○	○
4	○	○	○	○
5	○	○	○	○
6	○	○	○	○
7	○	○	○	○
8	○	○	○	○
9	○	○	○	○
10	○	○	○	○
11	○	○	○	○
12	○	○	○	○
13	○	○	○	○
14	○	○	○	○
15	○	○	○	○
16	○	○	○	○
17	○	○	○	○
18	○	○	○	○
19	○	○	○	○
20	○	○	○	○
21	○	○	○	○
22	○	○	○	○
23	○	○	○	○
24	○	○	○	○
25	○	○	○	○

Answers

1 Correct answer—**D**

D/A

$$0.6 \text{ g} \times \frac{1{,}000 \text{ mg}}{1 \text{ g}} = 600 \text{ mg}$$

R/P

$$1 \text{ g} : 1{,}000 \text{ mg} :: 0.6 \text{ g} : x \text{ mg}$$
$$x = 1{,}000 \times 0.6$$
$$x = 600 \text{ mg}$$

2 Correct answer—**B**

D/A

$$30 \text{ mg} \times \frac{1{,}000 \text{ mcg}}{1 \text{ mg}} = 30{,}000 \text{ mcg}$$

R/P

$$1 \text{ mg} : 1{,}000 \text{ mcg} :: 30 \text{ mg} : x \text{ mcg}$$
$$x = 1{,}000 \times 30$$
$$x = 30{,}000 \text{ mcg}$$

3 Correct answer—**C**

D/A

$$10 \text{ kg} \times \frac{1{,}000 \text{ g}}{1 \text{ kg}} = 10{,}000 \text{ g}$$

R/P

$$1 \text{ kg} : 1{,}000 \text{ g} :: 10 \text{ kg} : x \text{ g}$$
$$x = 1{,}000 \times 10$$
$$x = 10{,}000 \text{ g}$$

4 Correct answer—**B**

D/A

$$0.03 \text{ mg} \times \frac{1 \text{ g}}{1{,}000 \text{ mg}} = \frac{0.03 \text{ g}}{1{,}000} = 0.00003 \text{ g}$$

R/P

$$1{,}000 \text{ mg} : 1 \text{ g} :: 0.03 \text{ mg} : x \text{ g}$$
$$1{,}000x = 0.03$$
$$x = \frac{0.03}{1{,}000}$$
$$x = 0.00003 \text{ g}$$

5 Correct answer — **C**

D/A

$$0.75 \text{ g} \times \frac{1{,}000 \text{ mg}}{1 \text{ g}} = 750 \text{ mg}$$

R/P

$$1 \text{ g} : 1{,}000 \text{ mg} :: 0.75 \text{ g} : x \text{ mg}$$
$$x = 1{,}000 \times 0.75$$
$$x = 750 \text{ mg}$$

6 Correct answer — **C**

D/A

$$4.8 \text{ kg} \times \frac{1{,}000 \text{ g}}{1 \text{ kg}} = 4{,}800 \text{ g}$$

R/P

$$1 \text{ kg} : 1{,}000 \text{ g} :: 4.8 \text{ kg} : x \text{ g}$$
$$x = 1{,}000 \times 4.8$$
$$x = 4{,}800 \text{ g}$$

7 Correct answer — **A**

D/A

$$750 \text{ mg} \times \frac{1 \text{ g}}{1{,}000 \text{ mg}} = \frac{750 \text{ g}}{1{,}000} = 0.75 \text{ g}$$

R/P

$$1{,}000 \text{ mg} : 1 \text{ g} :: 750 \text{ mg} : x \text{ g}$$
$$1{,}000x = 750$$
$$x = \frac{750}{1{,}000}$$
$$x = 0.75 \text{ g}$$

8 Correct answer — **A**

D/A

$$0.0002 \text{ g} \times \frac{1{,}000 \text{ mg}}{1 \text{ g}} = 0.2 \text{ mg}$$

R/P

$$1 \text{ g} : 1{,}000 \text{ mg} :: 0.0002 \text{ g} : x \text{ mg}$$
$$x = 1{,}000 \times 0.0002$$
$$x = 0.2 \text{ mg}$$

9 Correct answer — **D**

D/A

$$0.2 \cancel{g} \times \frac{1,000 \text{ mg}}{1 \cancel{g}} = 200 \text{ mg}$$

R/P

$$1 \text{ g} : 1,000 \text{ mg} :: 0.2 \text{ g} : x \text{ mg}$$
$$x = 1,000 \times 0.2$$
$$x = 200 \text{ mg}$$

10 Correct answer — **C**

D/A

$$3 \cancel{g} \times \frac{1,000 \text{ mg}}{1 \cancel{g}} = 3,000 \text{ mg}$$

R/P

$$1 \text{ g} : 1,000 \text{ mg} :: 3 \text{ g} : x \text{ mg}$$
$$x = 1,000 \times 3$$
$$x = 3,000 \text{ mg}$$

11 Correct answer — **B**

D/A

$$0.004 \cancel{g} \times \frac{1,000 \text{ mg}}{1 \cancel{g}} = 4 \text{ mg}$$

R/P

$$1 \text{ g} : 1,000 \text{ mg} :: 0.004 \text{ g} : x \text{ mg}$$
$$x = 1,000 \times 0.004$$
$$x = 4 \text{ mg}$$

12 Correct answer — **C**

D/A

$$0.016 \cancel{\text{mg}} \times \frac{1,000 \text{ mcg}}{1 \cancel{\text{mg}}} = 16 \text{ mcg}$$

R/P

$$1 \text{ mg} : 1,000 \text{ mcg} :: 0.016 \text{ mg} : x \text{ mcg}$$
$$x = 1,000 \times 0.016$$
$$x = 16 \text{ mcg}$$

13 Correct answer — C

D/A

$$0.0003 \cancel{g} \times \frac{1{,}000 \text{ mg}}{1 \cancel{g}} = 0.3 \text{ mg}$$

R/P

1 g : 1,000 mg :: 0.0003 g : *x* mg
$$x = 1{,}000 \times 0.0003$$
$$x = 0.3 \text{ mg}$$

14 Correct answer — A

D/A

$$0.002 \cancel{mg} \times \frac{1{,}000 \text{ mcg}}{1 \cancel{mg}} = 2 \text{ mcg}$$

R/P

1 mg : 1,000 mcg :: 0.002 mg : *x* mcg
$$x = 1{,}000 \times 0.002$$
$$x = 2 \text{ mcg}$$

15 Correct answer — B

D/A

$$6 \cancel{kg} \times \frac{1{,}000 \text{ g}}{1 \cancel{kg}} = 6{,}000 \text{ g}$$

R/P

1 kg : 1,000 g :: 6 kg : *x* g
$$x = 1{,}000 \times 6$$
$$x = 6{,}000 \text{ g}$$

16 Correct answer — D

D/A

$$250 \cancel{mcg} \times \frac{1 \text{ mg}}{1{,}000 \cancel{mcg}} = \frac{250 \text{ mg}}{1{,}000} = 0.25 \text{ mg}$$

R/P

$$1,000 \text{ mcg} : 1 \text{ mg} :: 250 \text{ mcg} : x \text{ mg}$$
$$1,000x = 250$$
$$x = \frac{250}{1,000}$$
$$x = 0.25 \text{ mg}$$

17 Correct answer — **D**

D/A

$$2.5 \cancel{U} \times \frac{1,000 \text{ mU}}{1 \cancel{U}} = 2,500 \text{ mU}$$

R/P

$$1 \text{ U} : 1,000 \text{ mU} :: 2.5 \text{ U} : x \text{ mU}$$
$$x = 1,000 \times 2.5$$
$$x = 2,500 \text{ mU}$$

18 Correct answer — **A**

D/A

$$0.25 \text{ liter} \times \frac{1,000 \text{ ml}}{1 \text{ liter}} = 250 \text{ ml}$$

R/P

$$1 \text{ liter} : 1,000 \text{ ml} :: 0.25 \text{ liter} : x \text{ ml}$$
$$x = 1,000 \times 0.25$$
$$x = 250 \text{ ml}$$

19 Correct answer — **B**

D/A

$$300 \text{ mU} \times \frac{1 \text{ U}}{1,000 \text{ mU}} = \frac{300 \text{ U}}{1,000} = 0.3 \text{ U}$$

R/P

$$1,000 \text{ mU} : 1 \text{ U} :: 300 \text{ mU} : x \text{ U}$$
$$1,000x = 300$$
$$x = \frac{300}{1,000}$$
$$x = 0.3 \text{ U}$$

20 Correct answer — **D**

D/A

$$0.00065 \text{ g} \times \frac{1,000 \text{ mg}}{1 \text{ g}} = 0.65 \text{ mg}$$

R/P

$$1 \text{ g} : 1{,}000 \text{ mg} :: 0.00065 \text{ g} : x \text{ mg}$$
$$x = 1{,}000 \times 0.00065$$
$$x = 0.65 \text{ mg}$$

21 Correct answer — C

D/A

$$1 \text{ m\cancel{cg}} \times \frac{1 \text{ mg}}{1{,}000 \text{ m\cancel{cg}}} = \frac{1 \text{ mg}}{1{,}000} = 0.001 \text{ mg}$$

R/P

$$1{,}000 \text{ mcg} : 1 \text{ mg} :: 1 \text{ mcg} : x \text{ mg}$$
$$1000x = 1$$
$$x = \frac{1}{1{,}000}$$
$$x = 0.001 \text{ mg}$$

22 Correct answer — B

D/A

$$600 \text{ m\cancel{g}} \times \frac{1 \text{ g}}{1{,}000 \text{ m\cancel{g}}} = \frac{600 \text{ g}}{1{,}000} = 0.6 \text{ g}$$

R/P

$$1{,}000 \text{ mg} : 1 \text{ g} :: 600 \text{ mg} : x \text{ g}$$
$$1{,}000x = 600$$
$$x = \frac{600}{1{,}000}$$
$$x = 0.6 \text{ g}$$

23 Correct answer — C

D/A

$$0.25 \text{ m\cancel{g}} \times \frac{1{,}000 \text{ mcg}}{1 \text{ m\cancel{g}}} = 250 \text{ mcg}$$

R/P

$$1 \text{ mg} : 1{,}000 \text{ mcg} :: 0.25 \text{ mg} : x \text{ mcg}$$
$$x = 1{,}000 \times 0.25$$
$$x = 250 \text{ mcg}$$

24 Correct answer — D

D/A

$$300 \text{ m\cancel{g}} \times \frac{1 \text{ g}}{1{,}000 \text{ m\cancel{g}}} = \frac{300 \text{ g}}{1{,}000} = 0.3 \text{ g}$$

R/P

$$1{,}000 \text{ mg} : 1 \text{ g} :: 300 \text{ mg} : x \text{ g}$$
$$1{,}000x = 300$$
$$x = \frac{300}{1{,}000}$$
$$x = 0.3 \text{ g}$$

25 Correct answer—**A**

D/A

$$10 \text{ mg} \times \frac{1 \text{ g}}{1{,}000 \text{ mg}} = \frac{10 \text{ g}}{1{,}000} = 0.01 \text{ g}$$

R/P

$$1{,}000 \text{ mg} : 1 \text{ g} :: 10 \text{ mg} : x \text{ g}$$
$$1{,}000x = 10$$
$$x = \frac{10}{1{,}000}$$
$$x = 0.01 \text{ g}$$

CHAPTER 2

Apothecaries' and Household Systems

Questions

1 6 tsp equal how many tablespoons?

A. ½ Tbs
B. 2 Tbs
C. 3 Tbs
D. 4 Tbs

2 4 Tbs equal how many fluidounces?

A. 2 f℥
B. 6 f℥
C. 8 f℥
D. 12 f℥

3 ½ pt equals how many fluidounces?

A. 1 f℥
B. 2¼ f℥
C. 4 f℥
D. 8 f℥

4 f℥ xxiv equal how many pints?

A. 1¼ pt
B. 1½ pt
C. 3 pt
D. 4 pt

5 f℥ iss equal how many drops?

A. 24 gtt
B. 29 gtt
C. 60 gtt
D. 90 gtt

6 ¼ tsp equals how many drops?

A. 3 gtt
B. 9 gtt
C. 12 gtt
D. 15 gtt

7 3 Tbs equal how many teaspoons?

A. ⅓ tsp
B. 6 tsp
C. 9 tsp
D. 30 tsp

8 16 gtt equal how many minims?

A. ⅛ ℳ
B. 4 ℳ
C. 16 ℳ
D. 32 ℳ

9 ½ qt equals how many fluidounces?

A. 16 f℥
B. 32 f℥
C. 88 f℥
D. 500 f℥

10 f℥ iii equal how many fluidrams?

A. 3½ f℥
B. 10 f℥
C. 12 f℥
D. 24 f℥

11 How many pints are in 4 cups?

A. ½ pt
B. 2 pt
C. 16 pt
D. 24 pt

12 f℥ xvi equal how many fluidounces?

A. 2 f℥
B. 18 f℥
C. 23 f℥
D. 144 f℥

13 f℥ v equal how many tablespoons?

A. 10 Tbs
B. 42 Tbs
C. 65 Tbs
D. 81 Tbs

14 How many fluidounces are in 3 pt?

A. 9 f℥
B. 24 f℥
C. 48 f℥
D. 56 f℥

15 2 oz equal how many cups?

    A. ⅛ cup
    B. ¼ cup
    C. ½ cup
    D. 1 cup

16 How many teaspoons equal 30 ♍?

    A. ¼ tsp
    B. ⅓ tsp
    C. ½ tsp
    D. ¾ tsp

17 f℥ viii equal how many fluidrams?

    A. 8 f℈
    B. 29 f℈
    C. 48 f℈
    D. 64 f℈

18 f℥ xvi equal how many quarts?

    A. ¼ qt
    B. ½ qt
    C. 2 qt
    D. 18 qt

19 How many ounces are in 5 lb?

    A. 20 oz
    B. 66 oz
    C. 80 oz
    D. 97 oz

20 4 oz equal how many pounds?

    A. ¼ lb
    B. 1 lb
    C. 24 lb
    D. 48 lb

21 1½ tsp equal how many fluidrams?

    A. ½ f℈
    B. ¾ f℈
    C. 1½ f℈
    D. 2⅜ f℈

22 The physician writes an order for the cathartic magnesium hydroxide (Milk of Magnesia) f℥ xii. How many fluidounces does this equal?

A. ¼ f℥
B. 1½ f℥
C. 3¼ f℥
D. 5 f℥

23 The nurse prepares to administer a dose of 6 tsp of aluminum hydroxide gel (Amphojel). What is the equivalent dose in tablespoons?

A. 1½ Tbs
B. 2 Tbs
C. 2½ Tbs
D. 3 Tbs

Answer sheet

	A	B	C	D
1	○	○	○	○
2	○	○	○	○
3	○	○	○	○
4	○	○	○	○
5	○	○	○	○
6	○	○	○	○
7	○	○	○	○
8	○	○	○	○
9	○	○	○	○
10	○	○	○	○
11	○	○	○	○
12	○	○	○	○
13	○	○	○	○
14	○	○	○	○
15	○	○	○	○
16	○	○	○	○
17	○	○	○	○
18	○	○	○	○
19	○	○	○	○
20	○	○	○	○
21	○	○	○	○
22	○	○	○	○
23	○	○	○	○

Key: D/A = dimensional analysis
R/P = ratio and proportion

Answers

1 Correct answer — **B**

D/A

$$6 \text{ tsp} \times \frac{1 \text{ Tbs}}{3 \text{ tsp}} = \frac{6 \text{ Tbs}}{3} = 2 \text{ Tbs}$$

R/P

$$3 \text{ tsp} : 1 \text{ Tbs} :: 6 \text{ tsp} : x \text{ Tbs}$$
$$3x = 6$$
$$x = \frac{6}{3}$$
$$x = 2 \text{ Tbs}$$

2 Correct answer — **A**

D/A

$$4 \text{ Tbs} \times \frac{1 \text{ f}\mathrecipe}{2 \text{ Tbs}} = \frac{4 \text{ f}\mathrecipe}{2} = 2 \text{ f}\mathrecipe$$

R/P

$$2 \text{ Tbs} : 1 \text{ f}\mathrecipe :: 4 \text{ Tbs} : x \text{ f}\mathrecipe$$
$$2x = 4$$
$$x = \frac{4}{2}$$
$$x = 2 \text{ f}\mathrecipe$$

3 Correct answer — **D**

D/A

$$\tfrac{1}{2} \text{ pt} \times \frac{16 \text{ f}\mathrecipe}{1 \text{ pt}} = \frac{16 \text{ f}\mathrecipe}{2} = 8 \text{ f}\mathrecipe$$

R/P

$$1 \text{ pt} : 16 \text{ f}\mathrecipe :: \tfrac{1}{2} \text{ pt} : x \text{ f}\mathrecipe$$
$$x = 16 \times \tfrac{1}{2}$$
$$x = 8 \text{ f}\mathrecipe$$

4 Correct answer — **B**

D/A

$$24 \text{ f}\mathrecipe \times \frac{1 \text{ pt}}{16 \text{ f}\mathrecipe} = \frac{24 \text{ pt}}{16} = 1\tfrac{1}{2} \text{ pt}$$

R/P

$$16 \text{ f}\text{℥} : 1 \text{ pt} :: 24 \text{ f}\text{℥} : x \text{ pt}$$
$$16x = 24$$
$$x = \frac{24}{16}$$
$$x = 1\frac{1}{2} \text{ pt}$$

5 Correct answer—**D**

D/A

$$1.5 \text{ f}\text{℥} \times \frac{60 \text{ gtt}}{1 \text{ f}\text{℥}} = 90 \text{ gtt}$$

R/P

$$1 \text{ f}\text{℥} : 60 \text{ gtt} :: 1.5 \text{ f}\text{℥} : x \text{ gtt}$$
$$x = 60 \times 1.5$$
$$x = 90 \text{ gtt}$$

6 Correct answer—**D**

D/A

$$\frac{1}{4} \text{ tsp} \times \frac{60 \text{ gtt}}{1 \text{ tsp}} = \frac{60 \text{ gtt}}{4} = 15 \text{ gtt}$$

R/P

$$1 \text{ tsp} : 60 \text{ gtt} :: \frac{1}{4} \text{ tsp} : x \text{ gtt}$$
$$x = 60 \times \frac{1}{4}$$
$$x = 15 \text{ gtt}$$

7 Correct answer—**C**

D/A

$$3 \text{ Tbs} \times \frac{3 \text{ tsp}}{1 \text{ Tbs}} = 9 \text{ tsp}$$

R/P

$$1 \text{ Tbs} : 3 \text{ tsp} :: 3 \text{ Tbs} : x \text{ tsp}$$
$$x = 3 \times 3$$
$$x = 9 \text{ tsp}$$

8 Correct answer—**C**
Remember: gtt = ♏. This is an equivalent.

D/A

$$16 \text{ gtt} = 16 \text{ ♏}$$

R/P

$$16 \text{ gtt} = 16 \text{ ♏}$$

9 Correct answer — **A**

D/A

$$\frac{1}{2} \; \cancel{qt} \times \frac{32 \; f\text{℥}}{1 \; \cancel{qt}} = \frac{32 \; f\text{℥}}{2} = 16 \; f\text{℥}$$

R/P

$$1 \; qt : 32 \; f\text{℥} :: \tfrac{1}{2} \; qt : x \; f\text{℥}$$
$$x = 32 \times \tfrac{1}{2}$$
$$x = 16 \; f\text{℥}$$

10 Correct answer — **D**

D/A

$$3 \; \cancel{f\text{℥}} \times \frac{8 \; f\text{ʒ}}{1 \; \cancel{f\text{℥}}} = 24 \; f\text{ʒ}$$

R/P

$$1 \; f\text{℥} : 8 \; f\text{ʒ} :: 3 \; f\text{℥} : x \; f\text{ʒ}$$
$$x = 8 \times 3$$
$$x = 24 \; f\text{ʒ}$$

11 Correct answer — **B**

D/A

$$4 \; \cancel{cups} \times \frac{1 \; pt}{2 \; \cancel{cups}} = \frac{4 \; pt}{2} = 2 \; pt$$

R/P

$$2 \; cups : 1 \; pt :: 4 \; cups : x \; pt$$
$$2x = 4$$
$$x = \frac{4}{2}$$
$$x = 2 \; pt$$

12 Correct answer — **A**

D/A

$$16 \; \cancel{f\text{ʒ}} \times \frac{1 \; f\text{℥}}{8 \; \cancel{f\text{ʒ}}} = \frac{16 \; f\text{℥}}{8} = 2 \; f\text{℥}$$

R/P

$$8 \; f\text{ʒ} : 1 \; f\text{℥} :: 16 \; f\text{ʒ} : x \; f\text{℥}$$
$$8x = 16$$
$$x = \frac{16}{8}$$
$$x = 2 \; f\text{℥}$$

13 Correct answer — **A**

D/A

$$5 \text{ f} \text{ʒ} \times \frac{2 \text{ Tbs}}{1 \text{ fʒ}} = 10 \text{ Tbs}$$

R/P

$$1 \text{ fʒ} : 2 \text{ Tbs} :: 5 \text{ fʒ} : x \text{ Tbs}$$
$$x = 2 \times 5$$
$$x = 10 \text{ Tbs}$$

14 Correct answer — **C**

D/A

$$3 \text{ pt} \times \frac{16 \text{ fʒ}}{1 \text{ pt}} = 48 \text{ fʒ}$$

R/P

$$1 \text{ pt} : 16 \text{ fʒ} :: 3 \text{ pt} : x \text{ fʒ}$$
$$x = 16 \times 3$$
$$x = 48 \text{ fʒ}$$

15 Correct answer — **B**

D/A

$$2 \text{ fʒ} \times \frac{1 \text{ cup}}{8 \text{ fʒ}} = \frac{2 \text{ cups}}{8} = \tfrac{1}{4} \text{ cup}$$

R/P

$$8 \text{ fʒ} : 1 \text{ cup} :: 2 \text{ fʒ} : x \text{ cups}$$
$$8x = 2$$
$$x = \tfrac{2}{8}$$
$$x = \tfrac{1}{4} \text{ cup}$$

16 Correct answer — **C**

D/A

$$30 \text{ ♏} \times \frac{1 \text{ tsp}}{60 \text{ ♏}} = \frac{30 \text{ tsp}}{60} = \tfrac{1}{2} \text{ tsp}$$

R/P

$$60 \text{ ♏} : 1 \text{ tsp} :: 30 \text{ ♏} : x \text{ tsp}$$
$$60x = 30$$
$$x = \frac{30}{60}$$
$$x = \tfrac{1}{2} \text{ tsp}$$

17 Correct answer—D

D/A

$$8 \text{ f℥} \times \frac{8 \text{ fℨ}}{1 \text{ f℥}} = 64 \text{ fℨ}$$

R/P

$$1 \text{ fℨ} : 8 \text{ fℨ} :: 8 \text{ fℨ} : x \text{ fℨ}$$
$$x = 8 \times 8$$
$$x = 64 \text{ fℨ}$$

18 Correct answer—B

D/A

$$16 \text{ fℨ} \times \frac{1 \text{ qt}}{32 \text{ fℨ}} = \frac{16 \text{ qt}}{32} = \text{½ qt}$$

R/P

$$32 \text{ fℨ} : 1 \text{ qt} :: 16 \text{ fℨ} : x \text{ qt}$$
$$32x = 16$$
$$x = \frac{16}{32}$$
$$x = \text{½ qt}$$

19 Correct answer—C

D/A

$$5 \text{ lb} \times \frac{16 \text{ oz}}{1 \text{ lb}} = 80 \text{ oz}$$

R/P

$$1 \text{ lb} : 16 \text{ oz} :: 5 \text{ lb} : x \text{ oz}$$
$$x = 16 \times 5$$
$$x = 80 \text{ oz}$$

20 Correct answer—A

D/A

$$4 \text{ oz} \times \frac{1 \text{ lb}}{16 \text{ oz}} = \frac{4 \text{ lb}}{16} = \text{¼ lb}$$

R/P

$$16 \text{ oz} : 1 \text{ lb} :: 4 \text{ oz} : x \text{ lb}$$
$$16x = 4$$
$$x = \frac{4}{16}$$
$$x = \text{¼ lb}$$

21 Correct answer — **C**

Remember: tsp = f℥. This is an equivalent.

D/A
$$1\frac{1}{2} \text{ tsp} = 1\frac{1}{2} \text{ f℥}$$

R/P
$$1\frac{1}{2} \text{ tsp} = 1\frac{1}{2} \text{ f℥}$$

22 Correct answer — **B**

D/A
$$12 \text{ f℥} \times \frac{1 \text{ f℥}}{8 \text{ f℥}} = \frac{12 \text{ f℥}}{8} = 1\frac{1}{2} \text{ f℥}$$

R/P
$$8 \text{ f℥} : 1 \text{ f℥} :: 12 \text{ f℥} : x \text{ f℥}$$
$$8x = 12$$
$$x = \frac{12}{8}$$
$$x = 1\frac{1}{2} \text{ f℥}$$

23 Correct answer — **B**

D/A
$$6 \text{ tsp} \times \frac{1 \text{ Tbs}}{3 \text{ tsp}} = \frac{6 \text{ Tbs}}{3} = 2 \text{ Tbs}$$

R/P
$$3 \text{ tsp} : 1 \text{ Tbs} :: 6 \text{ tsp} : x \text{ Tbs}$$
$$3x = 6$$
$$x = \frac{6}{3}$$
$$x = 2 \text{ Tbs}$$

CHAPTER 3

Conversion Between Systems

Questions

1 1 gr = _____ mcg

A. 60
B. 100
C. 600
D. 60,000

2 5 lb = _____ g

A. 2,273
B. 3,114
C. 5,929
D. 18,038

3 0.1 mg = _____ g

A. $\frac{1}{6,000}$
B. $\frac{1}{600}$
C. $\frac{1}{100}$
D. $\frac{1}{30}$

4 $\frac{1}{6}$ gr = _____ mg

A. 10
B. 25
C. 250
D. 360

5 110 lb = _____ kg

A. 5
B. 50
C. 72
D. 76

6 2½ qt = _____ ml

A. 1,250
B. 2,500
C. 3,000
D. 45,000

7 75 ℳ = _____ ml

A. 2
B. 5
C. 10
D. 75

8 1,250 cc = _____ cups

 A. 1⅔
 B. 2½
 C. 3
 D. 5

9 480 ml = _____ f℥

 A. 4
 B. 6
 C. 16
 D. 24

10 0.4 g = _____ gr

 A. 1
 B. 2⅜
 C. 6
 D. 8

11 0.3 ml = _____ ♏

 A. 3
 B. 5
 C. 20
 D. 22

12 120 gtt = _____ Tbs

 A. ⅔
 B. ¾
 C. 8
 D. 12

13 10 lb = _____ g

 A. 44
 B. 460
 C. 4,545
 D. 45,455

14 f℥ v = _____ cc

 A. 50
 B. 125
 C. 150
 D. 160

15 1,500 g = _____ lb

    A. ⅛
    B. ⅖
    C. 2⅜
    D. 3⅓

16 5′ 6″ = _____ cm

    A. 84
    B. 165
    C. 190
    D. 210

17 3 gr = _____ g

    A. 0.1
    B. 0.2
    C. 0.8
    D. 1

18 2,500 mcg = _____ kg

    A. 0.00000019
    B. 0.00000025
    C. 0.0000025
    D. 0.00019

19 7½ gr = _____ g

    A. 0.5
    B. 0.7
    C. 12
    D. 90

20 1 teacup = _____ f℥

    A. 3½
    B. 4
    C. 48
    D. 97

21 5 gal = _____ cups

    A. 5
    B. 10
    C. 75
    D. 80

22 ¼ pt = _____ ml

A. 33
B. 75
C. 125
D. 500

23 105° F = _____ ° C

A. 31.9
B. 34.5
C. 39.8
D. 40.6

24 ¼₀₀ gr = _____ mg

A. 0.15
B. 0.25
C. 2
D. 150

25 1,000 mg = _____ gr

A. 15
B. 20
C. 25
D. 60

26 100 pt = _____ gal

A. 4
B. 12½
C. 25
D. 50

27 38° C = _____ ° F

A. 97.6
B. 99.4
C. 100.4
D. 101.7

28 750 gr = _____ g

A. 7.5
B. 40
C. 50
D. 450

29 50 ♏ = _____ ml

A. 1.25
B. 2.8
C. 3.3
D. 5

30 f℥ i = _____ ♏

A. 75
B. 225
C. 450
D. 1,000

31 600 mg = _____ gr

A. 10
B. 15
C. 250
D. 6,000

32 1.5 mg = _____ gr

A. $\frac{1}{300}$
B. $\frac{1}{40}$
C. $\frac{1}{12}$
D. 5

33 40 cm = _____ ″

A. 2¼
B. 8
C. 16
D. 20

34 0.08 mg = _____ gr

A. $\frac{1}{3,000}$
B. $\frac{1}{900}$
C. $\frac{1}{750}$
D. $\frac{1}{80}$

35 0.002 g = _____ gr

A. $\frac{1}{750}$
B. $\frac{3}{100}$
C. 20
D. 200

36 2.5 gal = _____ ml

A. 300
B. 750
C. 2,500
D. 10,000

37 70 kg = _____ lb

A. 96
B. 127
C. 154
D. 172

38 gr $\frac{1}{100}$ = _____ mcg

A. 600
B. 810
C. 2,974
D. 300,000

39 6 tsp = _____ f℥

A. ⅓
B. 1
C. 2
D. 30

40 100 ml = _____ pt

A. $\frac{1}{100}$
B. $\frac{1}{50}$
C. $\frac{1}{10}$
D. ⅕

41 6 ♏ = _____ ml

A. 0.4
B. 0.9
C. 1.6
D. 44

42 The physician orders 1,500 mg of ascorbic acid (vitamin C). What is the equivalent dose in grains?

A. $\frac{1}{25}$ gr
B. 2 gr
C. 25 gr
D. 125 gr

43 The physician orders phenobarbital (Luminal) 45 mg. How many grains are ordered?

A. ¾ gr
B. 3 gr
C. 10 gr
D. 24 gr

44 The nurse is preparing to administer 20 gtt of Lugol's solution to a patient. What is the equivalent dose in milliliters?

A. 0.6 ml
B. 1.3 ml
C. 3.2 ml
D. 8 ml

45 A patient's order reads: "Acetylsalicylic acid (aspirin) 15 gr stat." How many grams have been ordered?

A. 0.09 g
B. 0.4 g
C. 1 g
D. 1.5 g

46 The physician orders castor oil (Neoloid) ½ f℥. What is the equivalent dose in milliliters?

A. 0.125 ml
B. 2.5 ml
C. 7.5 ml
D. 15 ml

Answer sheet

	A	B	C	D			A	B	C	D
1	○	○	○	○		**31**	○	○	○	○
2	○	○	○	○		**32**	○	○	○	○
3	○	○	○	○		**33**	○	○	○	○
4	○	○	○	○		**34**	○	○	○	○
5	○	○	○	○		**35**	○	○	○	○
6	○	○	○	○		**36**	○	○	○	○
7	○	○	○	○		**37**	○	○	○	○
8	○	○	○	○		**38**	○	○	○	○
9	○	○	○	○		**39**	○	○	○	○
10	○	○	○	○		**40**	○	○	○	○
11	○	○	○	○		**41**	○	○	○	○
12	○	○	○	○		**42**	○	○	○	○
13	○	○	○	○		**43**	○	○	○	○
14	○	○	○	○		**44**	○	○	○	○
15	○	○	○	○		**45**	○	○	○	○
16	○	○	○	○		**46**	○	○	○	○
17	○	○	○	○						
18	○	○	○	○						
19	○	○	○	○						
20	○	○	○	○						
21	○	○	○	○						
22	○	○	○	○						
23	○	○	○	○						
24	○	○	○	○						
25	○	○	○	○						
26	○	○	○	○						
27	○	○	○	○						
28	○	○	○	○						
29	○	○	○	○						
30	○	○	○	○						

Answers

1 Correct answer — **D**
Remember: 1 gr = 60 mg

D/A

$$1 \ \cancel{gr} \times \frac{60 \ \cancel{mg}}{1 \ \cancel{gr}} \times \frac{1,000 \ mcg}{1 \ \cancel{mg}} = 60,000 \ mcg$$

R/P

$$1 \ mg : 1,000 \ mcg :: 60 \ mg : x \ mcg$$
$$x = 1,000 \times 60$$
$$x = 60,000 \ mcg$$

---

2 Correct answer — **A**

D/A

$$5 \ \cancel{lb} \times \frac{1 \ \cancel{kg}}{2.2 \ \cancel{lb}} \times \frac{1,000 \ g}{1 \ \cancel{kg}} = \frac{5,000 \ g}{2.2} = 2,272.7 \text{ or } 2,273 \ g$$

R/P

Step 1: Change pounds to kilograms.
$$2.2 \ lb : 1 \ kg :: 5 \ lb : x \ kg$$
$$2.2x = 5$$
$$x = \frac{5}{2.2}$$
$$x = 2.2727 \ kg$$

Step 2: Change kilograms to grams.
$$1 \ kg : 1,000 \ g :: 2.2727 \ kg : x \ g$$
$$x = 1,000 \times 2.2727$$
$$x = 2,272.7 \text{ or } 2,273 \ g$$

---

3 Correct answer — **B**

D/A

$$0.1 \ \cancel{mg} \times \frac{1 \ gr}{60 \ \cancel{mg}} = \frac{0.1 \ gr}{60} = \frac{1}{600} \ gr$$

R/P

$$60 \ mg : 1 \ gr :: 0.1 \ mg : x \ gr$$
$$60x = 0.1$$
$$x = \frac{0.1}{60}$$
$$x = \frac{1}{600} \ gr$$

4 Correct answer — **A**

D/A

$$\frac{1}{6} \text{ gr} \times \frac{60 \text{ mg}}{1 \text{ gr}} = \frac{60 \text{ mg}}{6} = 10 \text{ mg}$$

R/P

$$1 \text{ gr} : 60 \text{ mg} :: \frac{1}{6} \text{ gr} : x \text{ mg}$$
$$x = 60 \times \frac{1}{6}$$
$$x = 10 \text{ mg}$$

5 Correct answer — **B**

D/A

$$110 \text{ lb} \times \frac{1 \text{ kg}}{2.2 \text{ lb}} = \frac{110 \text{ kg}}{2.2} = 50 \text{ kg}$$

R/P

$$2.2 \text{ lb} : 1 \text{ kg} :: 110 \text{ lb} : x \text{ kg}$$
$$2.2x = 110$$
$$x = \frac{110}{2.2}$$
$$x = 50 \text{ kg}$$

6 Correct answer — **B**

D/A

$$\frac{5}{2} \text{ qt} \times \frac{1,000 \text{ ml}}{1 \text{ qt}} = \frac{5,000 \text{ ml}}{2} = 2,500 \text{ ml}$$

R/P

$$1 \text{ qt} : 1,000 \text{ ml} :: 2\frac{1}{2} \text{ qt} : x \text{ ml}$$
$$x = 1,000 \times 2.5$$
$$x = 2,500 \text{ ml}$$

7 Correct answer — **B**

D/A

$$75 \text{ m} \times \frac{1 \text{ ml}}{15 \text{ m}} = \frac{75 \text{ ml}}{15} = 5 \text{ ml}$$

R/P

$$15 \text{ m} : 1 \text{ ml} :: 75 \text{ m} : x \text{ ml}$$
$$15x = 75$$
$$x = \frac{75}{15}$$
$$x = 5 \text{ ml}$$

8 Correct answer—**D**

D/A

$$1{,}250 \text{ cc} \times \frac{1 \text{ cup}}{250 \text{ cc}} = \frac{1{,}250 \text{ cups}}{250} = 5 \text{ cups}$$

R/P

$$250 \text{ cc} : 1 \text{ cup} :: 1{,}250 \text{ cc} : x \text{ cups}$$
$$250x = 1{,}250$$
$$x = \frac{1{,}250}{250}$$
$$x = 5 \text{ cups}$$

9 Correct answer—**C**

D/A

$$480 \text{ ml} \times \frac{1 \text{ f℥}}{30 \text{ ml}} = \frac{480 \text{ f℥}}{30} = 16 \text{ f℥}$$

R/P

$$30 \text{ ml} : 1 \text{ f℥} :: 480 \text{ ml} : x \text{ f℥}$$
$$30x = 480$$
$$x = \frac{480}{30}$$
$$x = 16 \text{ f℥}$$

10 Correct answer—**C**

D/A

$$0.4 \text{ g} \times \frac{15 \text{ gr}}{1 \text{ g}} = 6 \text{ gr}$$

R/P

$$1 \text{ g} : 15 \text{ gr} :: 0.4 \text{ g} : x \text{ gr}$$
$$x = 15 \times 0.4$$
$$x = 6 \text{ gr}$$

11 Correct answer—**B**

D/A

$$0.3 \text{ ml} \times \frac{15 \text{ ℳ}}{1 \text{ ml}} = 4.5 \text{ or } 5 \text{ ℳ}$$

R/P

$$1 \text{ ml} : 15 \text{ ℳ} :: 0.3 \text{ ml} : x \text{ ℳ}$$
$$x = 15 \times 0.3$$
$$x = 4.5 \text{ or } 5 \text{ ℳ}$$

12 Correct answer — **A**

D/A

$$120 \text{ g\cancel{tt}} \times \frac{1 \text{ \cancel{tsp}}}{60 \text{ g\cancel{tt}}} \times \frac{1 \text{ Tbs}}{3 \text{ \cancel{tsp}}} = \frac{120 \text{ Tbs}}{180} = \text{⅔ Tbs}$$

R/P

Step 1: Change drops to teaspoons.
$$60 \text{ gtt} : 1 \text{ tsp} :: 120 \text{ gtt} : x \text{ tsp}$$
$$60x = 120$$
$$x = \frac{120}{60}$$
$$x = 2 \text{ tsp}$$

Step 2: Change teaspoons to tablespoons.
$$3 \text{ tsp} : 1 \text{ Tbs} :: 2 \text{ tsp} : x \text{ Tbs}$$
$$3x = 2$$
$$x = \text{⅔ Tbs}$$

13 Correct answer — **C**
Remember: 1,000 g = 1 kg

D/A

$$10 \text{ \cancel{lb}} \times \frac{1 \text{ \cancel{kg}}}{2.2 \text{ \cancel{lb}}} \times \frac{1{,}000 \text{ g}}{1 \text{ \cancel{kg}}} = \frac{10{,}000 \text{ g}}{2.2} = 4{,}545.4 \text{ or } 4{,}545 \text{ g}$$

R/P

$$2.2 \text{ lb} : 1{,}000 \text{ g} :: 10 \text{ lb} : x \text{ g}$$
$$2.2x = 10{,}000$$
$$x = \frac{10{,}000}{2.2}$$
$$x = 4{,}545.5 \text{ or } 4{,}545 \text{ g}$$

14 Correct answer — **C**

D/A

$$5 \text{ f\cancel{з}} \times \frac{30 \text{ cc}}{1 \text{ f\cancel{з}}} = 150 \text{ cc}$$

R/P

$$1 \text{ fз} : 30 \text{ cc} :: 5 \text{ fз} : x \text{ cc}$$
$$x = 30 \times 5$$
$$x = 150 \text{ cc}$$

15 Correct answer — **D**

D/A

$$1{,}500 \; \cancel{g} \times \frac{1 \; \cancel{kg}}{1{,}000 \; \cancel{g}} \times \frac{2.2 \; lb}{1 \; \cancel{kg}} = \frac{3{,}300 \; lb}{1{,}000} = 3.3 \; or \; 3\tfrac{1}{3} \; lb$$

R/P

Step 1: Change grams to kilograms.

$$1{,}000 \; g : 1 \; kg :: 1{,}500 \; g : x \; kg$$
$$1{,}000x = 1{,}500$$
$$x = \frac{1{,}500}{1{,}000}$$
$$x = 1.5 \; kg$$

Step 2: Change kilograms to pounds.

$$1 \; kg : 2.2 \; lb :: 1.5 \; kg : x \; lb$$
$$x = 2.2 \times 1.5$$
$$x = 3.3 \; or \; 3\tfrac{1}{3} \; lb$$

16 Correct answer — **B**

D/A

$$66'' \times \frac{2.5 \; cm}{1''} = 165 \; cm$$

R/P

$$1'' : 2.5 \; cm :: 66'' : x \; cm$$
$$x = 2.5 \times 66$$
$$x = 165 \; cm$$

17 Correct answer — **B**

D/A

$$3 \; \cancel{gr} \times \frac{1 \; g}{15 \; \cancel{gr}} = \frac{3 \; g}{15} = 0.2 \; g$$

R/P

$$15 \; gr : 1 \; g :: 3 \; gr : x \; g$$
$$15x = 3$$
$$x = \frac{3}{15}$$
$$x = 0.2 \; g$$

18 Correct answer — **C**

D/A

$$2,500 \; \text{mcg} \times \frac{1 \; \text{mg}}{1,000 \; \text{mcg}} \times \frac{1 \; \text{g}}{1,000 \; \text{mg}} \times \frac{1 \; \text{kg}}{1,000 \; \text{g}} =$$

$$\frac{25 \; \text{kg}}{10,000,000} = 0.0000025 \; \text{kg}$$

R/P

Step 1: Change micrograms to milligrams.

$$1,000 \; \text{mcg} : 1 \; \text{mg} :: 2,500 \; \text{mcg} : x \; \text{mg}$$
$$1,000x = 2,500$$
$$x = \frac{2,500}{1,000}$$
$$x = 2.5 \; \text{mg}$$

Step 2: Change milligrams to grams.

$$1,000 \; \text{mg} : 1 \; \text{g} :: 2.5 \; \text{mg} : x \; \text{g}$$
$$1,000x = 2.5$$
$$x = \frac{2.5}{1,000}$$
$$x = 0.0025 \; \text{g}$$

Step 3: Change grams to kilograms.

$$1,000 \; \text{g} : 1 \; \text{kg} :: 0.0025 \; \text{g} : x \; \text{kg}$$
$$1,000x = 0.0025$$
$$x = \frac{0.0025}{1,000}$$
$$x = 0.0000025 \; \text{kg}$$

19 Correct answer — **A**

Remember: $7\frac{1}{2}$ gr $= 0.5$ g

D/A

$$7.5 \; \text{gr} \times \frac{1 \; \text{g}}{15 \; \text{gr}} = \frac{7.5 \; \text{g}}{15} = 0.5 \; \text{g}$$

R/P

$$15 \; \text{gr} : 1 \; \text{g} :: 7\frac{1}{2} \; \text{gr} : x \; \text{g}$$
$$15x = 7.5$$
$$x = \frac{7.5}{15}$$
$$x = 0.5 \; \text{g}$$

20 Correct answer—**C**

Remember: 1 teacup = 6 f℥

D/A

$$1 \text{ teacup} \times \frac{6 \text{ f℥}}{1 \text{ teacup}} \times \frac{8 \text{ f℥}}{1 \text{ f℥}} = 48 \text{ f℥}$$

R/P

$$1 \text{ f℥} : 8 \text{ f℥} :: 6 \text{ f℥} : x \text{ f℥}$$
$$x = 8 \times 6$$
$$x = 48 \text{ f℥}$$

21 Correct answer—**D**

D/A

$$5 \text{ gal} \times \frac{4 \text{ qt}}{1 \text{ gal}} \times \frac{4 \text{ cups}}{1 \text{ qt}} = 80 \text{ cups}$$

R/P

Step 1: Change gallons to quarts.
$$1 \text{ gal} : 4 \text{ qt} :: 5 \text{ gal} : x \text{ qt}$$
$$x = 4 \times 5$$
$$x = 20 \text{ qt}$$
Step 2: Change quarts to cups.
$$1 \text{ qt} : 4 \text{ cups} :: 20 \text{ qt} : x \text{ cups}$$
$$x = 20 \times 4$$
$$x = 80 \text{ cups}$$

22 Correct answer—**C**

D/A

$$\tfrac{1}{4} \text{ pt} \times \frac{500 \text{ ml}}{1 \text{ pt}} = \frac{500 \text{ ml}}{4} = 125 \text{ ml}$$

R/P

$$1 \text{ pt} : 500 \text{ ml} :: \tfrac{1}{4} \text{ pt} : x \text{ ml}$$
$$x = 500 \times \tfrac{1}{4}$$
$$x = 125 \text{ ml}$$

23 Correct answer—**D**

Remember: This is the standard formula.

D/A

$$\frac{^\circ\text{F} - 32}{1.8} = {^\circ}\text{C}$$

$$\frac{105 - 32}{1.8} = \frac{73}{1.8} = 40.6^\circ \text{ C}$$

24

Correct answer — **A**

D/A

$$\frac{1 \text{ gr}}{400} \times \frac{60 \text{ mg}}{1 \text{ gr}} = \frac{6 \text{ mg}}{40} = 0.15 \text{ mg}$$

R/P

$$1 \text{ gr} : 60 \text{ mg} :: \frac{1}{400} \text{ gr} : x \text{ mg}$$
$$x = 60 \times \frac{1}{400}$$
$$x = 0.15 \text{ mg}$$

25

Correct answer — **A**

Remember: 1,000 mg = 15 gr

D/A

$$1{,}000 \text{ mg} \times \frac{1 \text{ g}}{1{,}000 \text{ mg}} \times \frac{15 \text{ gr}}{1 \text{ g}} = 15 \text{ gr}$$

R/P

$$1{,}000 \text{ mg} = 15 \text{ gr}$$

26

Correct answer — **B**

D/A

$$100 \text{ pt} \times \frac{1 \text{ qt}}{2 \text{ pt}} \times \frac{1 \text{ gal}}{4 \text{ qt}} = \frac{100 \text{ gal}}{8} = 12\frac{1}{2} \text{ gal}$$

R/P

Step 1: Change pints to quarts.

$$2 \text{ pt} : 1 \text{ qt} :: 100 \text{ pt} : x \text{ qt}$$
$$2x = 100$$
$$x = \frac{100}{2}$$
$$x = 50 \text{ qt}$$

Step 2: Change quarts to gallons.

$$4 \text{ qt} : 1 \text{ gal} :: 50 \text{ qt} : x \text{ gal}$$
$$4x = 50$$
$$x = \frac{50}{4}$$
$$x = 12\frac{1}{2} \text{ gal}$$

27 Correct answer — **C**

Remember: This is the standard formula.

D/A

$$(\degree C \times 1.8) + 32 = \degree F$$
$$(38 \times 1.8) + 32 = 100.4\degree\ F$$

28 Correct answer — **C**

D/A

$$750\ \text{gr} \times \frac{1\ g}{15\ \text{gr}} = \frac{750\ g}{15} = 50\ g$$

R/P

$$15\ gr : 1\ g :: 750\ gr : x\ g$$
$$15x = 750$$
$$x = \frac{750}{15}$$
$$x = 50\ g$$

29 Correct answer — **C**

D/A

$$50\ \text{m} \times \frac{1\ ml}{15\ \text{m}} = \frac{50\ ml}{15} = 3.3\ ml$$

R/P

$$15\ \text{m} : 1\ ml :: 50\ \text{m} : x\ ml$$
$$15x = 50$$
$$x = \frac{50}{15}$$
$$x = 3.3\ ml$$

30 Correct answer — **C**

Remember: f℥ = 30 ml

D/A

$$1\ \text{f℥} \times \frac{30\ ml}{1\ \text{f℥}} \times \frac{15\ \text{m}}{1\ ml} = 450\ \text{m}$$

R/P

$$1\ ml : 15\ \text{m} :: 30\ ml : x\ \text{m}$$
$$x = 15 \times 30$$
$$x = 450\ \text{m}$$

31 Correct answer — **A**

D/A

$$600 \text{ mg} \times \frac{1 \text{ gr}}{60 \text{ mg}} = 10 \text{ gr}$$

R/P

$$60 \text{ mg} : 1 \text{ gr} :: 600 \text{ mg} : x \text{ gr}$$
$$60x = 600$$
$$x = \frac{600}{60}$$
$$x = 10 \text{ gr}$$

32 Correct answer — **B**

D/A

$$1.5 \text{ mg} \times \frac{1 \text{ gr}}{60 \text{ mg}} = \frac{1.5 \text{ gr}}{60} = \frac{1}{40} \text{ gr}$$

R/P

$$60 \text{ mg} : 1 \text{ gr} :: 1.5 \text{ mg} : x \text{ gr}$$
$$60x = 1.5$$
$$x = \frac{1.5}{60}$$
$$x = \frac{1}{40} \text{ gr}$$

33 Correct answer — **C**

D/A

$$40 \text{ cm} \times \frac{1''}{2.5 \text{ cm}} = \frac{40''}{2.5} = 16''$$

R/P

$$2.5 \text{ cm} : 1'' :: 40 \text{ cm} : x''$$
$$2.5x = 40$$
$$x = \frac{40}{2.5}$$
$$x = 16''$$

34 Correct answer — C

D/A

$$0.08 \text{ mg} \times \frac{1 \text{ gr}}{60 \text{ mg}} = \frac{0.08 \text{ gr}}{60} = \text{1/750 gr}$$

R/P

$$60 \text{ mg} : 1 \text{ gr} :: 0.08 \text{ mg} : x \text{ gr}$$
$$60x = 0.08$$
$$x = \frac{0.08}{60}$$
$$x = \text{1/750 gr}$$

35 Correct answer — B

D/A

$$0.002 \text{ g} \times \frac{15 \text{ gr}}{1 \text{ g}} = 0.03 \text{ gr} = \text{3/100 gr}$$

R/P

$$1 \text{ g} : 15 \text{ gr} :: 0.002 \text{ g} : x \text{ gr}$$
$$x = 15 \times 0.002$$
$$x = 0.03 \text{ gr}$$
$$x = \text{3/100 gr}$$

36 Correct answer — D

D/A

$$2.5 \text{ gal} \times \frac{4 \text{ qt}}{1 \text{ gal}} \times \frac{1,000 \text{ ml}}{1 \text{ qt}} = 10,000 \text{ ml}$$

R/P

Step 1: Change gallons to quarts.
$$1 \text{ gal} : 4 \text{ qt} :: 2.5 \text{ gal} : x \text{ qt}$$
$$x = 4 \times 2.5$$
$$x = 10 \text{ qt}$$

Step 2: Change quarts to milliliters.
$$1 \text{ qt} : 1,000 \text{ ml} :: 10 \text{ qt} : x \text{ ml}$$
$$x = 1,000 \times 10$$
$$x = 10,000 \text{ ml}$$

37 Correct answer — C

D/A

$$70 \text{ kg} \times \frac{2.2 \text{ lb}}{1 \text{ kg}} = 154 \text{ lb}$$

R/P

$$1 \text{ kg} : 2.2 \text{ lb} :: 70 \text{ kg} : x \text{ lb}$$
$$x = 2.2 \times 70$$
$$x = 154 \text{ lb}$$

38 Correct answer — **A**

D/A

$$\frac{1 \text{ gr}}{100} \times \frac{60 \text{ mg}}{1 \text{ gr}} \times \frac{1{,}000 \text{ mcg}}{1 \text{ mg}} = \frac{60{,}000 \text{ mcg}}{100} = 600 \text{ mcg}$$

R/P

Step 1: Change grains to milligrams.
$$1 \text{ gr} : 60 \text{ mg} :: \frac{1}{100} \text{ gr} : x \text{ mg}$$
$$x = 60 \times \frac{1}{100}$$
$$x = 0.6 \text{ mg}$$

Step 2: Change milligrams to micrograms.
$$1 \text{ mg} : 1{,}000 \text{ mcg} :: 0.6 \text{ mg} : x \text{ mcg}$$
$$x = 1{,}000 \times 0.6$$
$$x = 600 \text{ mcg}$$

39 Correct answer — **B**

Remember: 2 Tbs = 1 f℥

D/A

$$6 \text{ tsp} \times \frac{1 \text{ Tbs}}{3 \text{ tsp}} \times \frac{1 \text{ f℥}}{2 \text{ Tbs}} = \frac{6 \text{ f℥}}{6} = 1 \text{ f℥}$$

R/P

$$3 \text{ tsp} : 1 \text{ Tbs} :: 6 \text{ tsp} : x \text{ Tbs}$$
$$3x = 6$$
$$x = \frac{6}{3}$$
$$x = 2 \text{ Tbs} = 1 \text{ f℥}$$

40 Correct answer — **D**

D/A

$$100 \text{ ml} \times \frac{1 \text{ pt}}{500 \text{ ml}} = \frac{100 \text{ pt}}{500} = \frac{1}{5} \text{ pt}$$

R/P

$$500 \text{ ml} : 1 \text{ pt} :: 100 \text{ ml} : x \text{ pt}$$
$$500x = 100$$
$$x = \frac{100}{500}$$
$$x = \frac{1}{5} \text{ pt}$$

41
Correct answer — **A**

D/A

$$6 \ \cancel{m} \times \frac{1 \ ml}{15 \ \cancel{m}} = \frac{6 \ ml}{15} = 0.4 \ ml$$

R/P

$$15 \ m : 1 \ ml :: 6 \ m : x \ ml$$
$$15x = 6$$
$$x = \frac{6}{15}$$
$$x = 0.4 \ ml$$

42
Correct answer — **C**

D/A

$$1{,}500 \ \cancel{mg} \times \frac{1 \ gr}{60 \ \cancel{mg}} = \frac{1{,}500 \ gr}{60} = 25 \ gr$$

R/P

$$60 \ mg : 1 \ gr :: 1{,}500 \ mg : x \ gr$$
$$60x = 1{,}500$$
$$x = \frac{1{,}500}{60}$$
$$x = 25 \ gr$$

43
Correct answer — **A**

D/A

$$45 \ \cancel{mg} \times \frac{1 \ gr}{60 \ \cancel{mg}} = \frac{45 \ gr}{60} = \tfrac{3}{4} \ gr$$

R/P

$$60 \ mg : 1 \ gr :: 45 \ mg : x \ gr$$
$$60x = 45$$
$$x = \frac{45}{60}$$
$$x = \tfrac{3}{4} \ gr$$

44
Correct answer — **B**

D/A

$$20 \ \cancel{gtt} \times \frac{1 \ ml}{15 \ gtt} = \frac{20 \ ml}{15} = 1.3 \ ml$$

R/P

$$15 \text{ gtt} : 1 \text{ ml} :: 20 \text{ gtt} : x \text{ ml}$$
$$15x = 20$$
$$x = \frac{20}{15}$$
$$x = 1.3 \text{ ml}$$

45 Correct answer — **C**

D/A

$$15 \text{ gr} = 1 \text{ g}$$

R/P

$$15 \text{ gr} = 1 \text{ g}$$

46 Correct answer — **D**

D/A

$$\frac{1}{2} \; f\!\cancel{\text{Ʒ}} \times \frac{30 \text{ ml}}{1 \; \cancel{f\text{Ʒ}}} = \frac{30 \text{ ml}}{2} = 15 \text{ ml}$$

R/P

$$1 \text{ f}\text{Ʒ} : 30 \text{ ml} :: \tfrac{1}{2} \text{ f}\text{Ʒ} : x \text{ ml}$$
$$x = 30 \times \tfrac{1}{2}$$
$$x = 15 \text{ ml}$$

CHAPTER 4

Nonparenteral Medications

Questions

1 The physician orders the anticonvulsant phenytoin (Dilantin) in an oral suspension 0.1 g P.O. The pharmacy sends up a bottle labeled 125 mg in 5 ml. How many milliliters should the nurse administer?

A. 0.4 ml
B. 4 ml
C. 15 ml
D. 27 ml

2 The physician orders digoxin (Lanoxin) elixir 0.25 mg. The bottle is labeled 0.05 mg/ml. How many milliliters are needed?

A. 5 ml
B. 10 ml
C. 30 ml
D. 35 ml

3 An antihypertensive agent, minoxidil (Loniten) 5 mg P.O., is ordered. Available tablets are labeled 2.5 mg each. How many tablets should be administered?

A. ½ tablet
B. 1 tablet
C. 2 tablets
D. 2¾ tablets

4 The physician orders 1,000 mg of acetaminophen (Tylenol) P.O. The only available tablets are 0.5 g each. How many tablets are needed to administer this dose?

A. 2 tablets
B. 10 tablets
C. 12 tablets
D. 14 tablets

5 The expectorant guaifenesin (Robitussin) 300 mg P.O. has been ordered. The bottle is labeled 100 mg = 5 ml. How many milliliters must be prepared?

A. 0.25 ml
B. 1 ml
C. 10 ml
D. 15 ml

6 The nurse prepares to administer an order for methocarbamol (Robaxin) 1.5 g P.O.; 500-mg tablets are available. How many tablets of this skeletal muscle relaxant should be administered?

A. 1¼ tablets
B. 2¼ tablets
C. 3 tablets
D. 4 tablets

7 The physician has ordered the sedative-hypnotic triazolam (Halcion) 0.25 mg P.O. The pharmacy sends a supply of 0.125-mg tablets. How many tablets should be administered?

A. 1 tablet
B. 2 tablets
C. 2½ tablets
D. 4 tablets

8 The antihypertensive captopril (Capoten) 50 mg P.O. has been ordered. Available tablets are labeled 12.5 mg each. How many tablets should be administered?

A. 4 tablets
B. 6 tablets
C. 8 tablets
D. 10 tablets

9 The physician has ordered 300 mg P.O. of the liquid form of the sedative-hypnotic chloral hydrate (Noctec). The bottle is labeled 500 mg = 5 ml. How many milliliters must be prepared?

A. 3 ml
B. 21 ml
C. 25 ml
D. 30 ml

10 The nurse is ordered to administer nystatin suspension (Mycostatin) 400,000 U to a patient. This antifungal drug arrives from the pharmacy in a bottle labeled 5 ml = 500,000 U. How many milliliters should be administered?

A. 4 ml
B. 8 ml
C. 8.2 ml
D. 20 ml

11 The physician orders a glucose tolerance test for a pregnant patient. The nurse is instructed to administer 25 g of glucose P.O. The only available glucose solution is labeled 50%. How many milliliters should be administered?

A. 20 ml
B. 50 ml
C. 100 ml
D. 150 ml

12 A patient is scheduled to receive 0.8 g P.O. of the analgesic ibuprofen (Motrin) t.i.d. Each tablet is labeled 400 mg. How many tablets should the nurse administer with each dose?

A. ½ tablet
B. 1 tablet
C. 2 tablets
D. 3 tablets

13 A patient is to receive 12 mg P.O. of the antineoplastic chlorambucil (Leukeran) daily, in divided doses. The label reads 1 tablet = 2 mg. How many tablets should be given daily?

A. ¾ tablet
B. 2 tablets
C. 4 tablets
D. 6 tablets

14 Phenobarbital (Luminal) 3 gr P.O. has been ordered for bedtime sedation. Tablets are 100 mg each. How many tablets are needed for this order?

A. ½ tablet
B. ¾ tablet
C. 2 tablets
D. 4 tablets

15 The physician has ordered colchicine (Colsalide), an antigout medication, 1.2 mg P.O. daily on a prophylactic basis. Available tablets are 600 mcg each. How many tablets should be given daily?

A. 2 tablets
B. 3 tablets
C. 10 tablets
D. 15 tablets

16 Levodopa (Larodopa) 2,000 mg P.O. has been ordered. This antiparkinsonian agent is available in 500-mg tablets. How many tablets should be administered?

A. 2 tablets
B. 4 tablets
C. 6 tablets
D. 18 tablets

17 The nurse transcribes an oral order for codeine ⅙ gr P.O. The pharmacy sends up 5-mg tablets. How many tablets should be prepared?

A. ¼ tablet
B. ½ tablet
C. 1½ tablets
D. 2 tablets

18 A patient is to receive 0.25 mg P.O. of digoxin (Lanoxin). The bottle is labeled 1 ml = 50 mcg. How many milliliters of this antiarrhythmic should be administered?

A. 0.005 ml
B. 0.5 ml
C. 5 ml
D. 50 ml

19 Saturated solution of potassium iodide (SSKI) 5 gtt has been ordered for a patient. How many milliliters of this expectorant should the nurse administer?

A. 0.125 ml
B. 0.25 ml
C. 0.3 ml
D. 0.75 ml

20 Opium tincture 0.2 ml via nasogastric tube has been ordered prophylactically to treat diarrhea. How many drops should be administered?

A. 3 gtt
B. 10 gtt
C. 12 gtt
D. 20 gtt

21 The anticholinergic belladonna leaf (Belladonna Tincture USP) 8 gtt P.O. has been ordered. How many minims should be given to the patient?

A. 8 ℥
B. 40 ℥
C. 45 ℥
D. 100 ℥

22 Amobarbital (Amytal) 0.1 g P.O. has been ordered. Available tablets for this sedative are labeled as 50 mg each. How many tablets are needed?

A. ¼ tablet
B. ½ tablet
C. 2 tablets
D. 4 tablets

23 The physician orders ascorbic acid (vitamin C) 1.5 g P.O. Tablets on hand are 500 mg each. How many tablets should be given?

A. ½ tablet
B. 1 tablet
C. 2 tablets
D. 3 tablets

24 The physician orders the antihypertensive clonidine (Catapres) 1.2 mg P.O. as a daily dose. Unit tablets available from the pharmacy are listed as 0.3 mg each. How many tablets should be given?

A. ½ tablet
B. 1 tablet
C. 4 tablets
D. 8 tablets

25 The hormone norethindrone (Norlutin) 10 mg P.O. has been ordered for a patient. Available tablets are labeled as 2.5 mg each. How many tablets should be administered?

A. 1 tablet
B. 2½ tablets
C. 3 tablets
D. 4 tablets

26 A physician orders methsuximide (Celontin Kapseals), an anticonvulsant drug, 1.2 g P.O. in divided doses. If each capsule contains 300 mg, how many capsules equal 1.2 g?

A. ½ capsule
B. ¾ capsule
C. 3 capsules
D. 4 capsules

27 The physician orders 8 mg of dexamethasone (Decadron) oral solution. The bottle is labeled 0.5 mg/0.5 ml. How many milliliters of this anti-inflammatory drug should be administered?

A. 1 ml
B. 2 ml
C. 8 ml
D. 16 ml

28 Dimenhydrinate (Dramamine) 50 mg P.O. is ordered for vomiting. The bottle is labeled 12.5 mg/4 ml. How many milliliters must be prepared?

A. 16 ml
B. 20 ml
C. 40 ml
D. 50 ml

29 The physician orders scopolamine 1 mg P.O. This anticholinergic drug is available in capsules of 0.25 mg each. How many capsules should be given?

A. 1 capsule
B. 2 capsules
C. 3 capsules
D. 4 capsules

30 The physician orders the thyroid hormone levothyroxine (Synthroid) 0.1 mg P.O. for a patient. Each tablet is 50 mcg. How many tablets should be prepared?

A. 1 tablet
B. 2 tablets
C. 4 tablets
D. None of the above

31 Calcium lactate 1.3 g P.O. has been ordered. The pharmacy sends up unit tablets of 325 mg each. How many tablets of this calcium supplement equal 1.3 g?

A. 2 tablets
B. 4 tablets
C. 10 tablets
D. None of the above

32 The physician has ordered 1,000,000 U of penicillin G potassium (Pentids) in an oral suspension. This antibiotic agent is labeled as 5 ml = 200,000 U. How many milliliters must be prepared?

A. 1 ml
B. 20 ml
C. 25 ml
D. 50 ml

33 Nystatin oral suspension 600,000 U is ordered. The bottle is labeled 1 ml = 100,000 U. How many milliliters of this antifungal agent should be administered?

A. 6 ml
B. 10 ml
C. 60 ml
D. 100 ml

34 Magnesium hydroxide (Milk of Magnesia) f℥ ii is ordered. How many milliliters of this laxative should be given?

A. 0.1 ml
B. 6 ml
C. 10 ml
D. 60 ml

35 The physician orders 5 ml of the stimulant laxative cascara sagrada. How many teaspoons must be administered?

A. ½ tsp
B. 1 tsp
C. 2¼ tsp
D. 3 tsp

36 The physician orders maltodextrin (Sumacal) 400 calories. The carbohydrate supplement powder is labeled 3.8 calories/g. How many grams will provide 400 calories?

A. 0.25 g
B. 0.75 g
C. 15 g
D. 105 g

37 A concentrated nutrition product (Sustacal HC) for tube feeding has been ordered at 80 calories/hour. Each 250-ml can is labeled 1.5 calories/ml. How many milliliters will provide 80 calories?

A. 53 ml
B. 80 ml
C. 114 ml
D. 290 ml

38 An 18-year-old female patient with hyperthyroidism is to receive 0.3 g P.O. of propylthiouracil (Propyl-Thyracil) daily. Available tablets are 50 mg each. How many tablets are needed for each dose?

A. 2 tablets
B. 6 tablets
C. 10 tablets
D. 12 tablets

39 The physician orders maprotiline hydrochloride (Ludiomil) 225 mg P.O. Available tablets of this tricyclic antidepressant are 75 mg each. How many tablets should be administered?

A. 1 tablet
B. 1½ tablets
C. 2 tablets
D. 3 tablets

40 An antibiotic, dicloxacillin sodium (Dynapen) 0.5 g P.O., has been ordered. The label on the bottle of oral suspension reads 62.5 mg/ml. How many milliliters must be administered?

A. 3 ml
B. 4.5 ml
C. 7 ml
D. 8 ml

41 A patient is to receive the antihypertensive drug labetalol (Normodyne) P.O. Each tablet equals 100 mg. If the maintenance dose is 0.4 g, how many tablets should be administered?

A. 4 tablets
B. 9 tablets
C. 10 tablets
D. 14 tablets

42 The laxative lactulose (Cephulac) has been ordered for a patient with partial systemic encephalopathy. The order is 30 g P.O. t.i.d. If this oral solution is labeled 10 g/15 ml, how many milliliters must the patient receive at each dose?

A. 0.25 ml
B. 1.2 ml
C. 7.5 ml
D. 45 ml

43 If the physician orders the hypoglycemic acetohexamide (Dymelor) 1 g P.O. and each tablet contains 250 mg, how many tablets should be given?

A. ¼ tablet
B. 2 tablets
C. 4 tablets
D. 6 tablets

44 The physician orders 200 mg P.O. of amantadine hydrochloride (Symmetrel), an antiviral and antiparkinsonian agent. The bottle is labeled 50 mg = 5 ml. How many fluidrams must be administered?

A. 4 f𝟛
B. 10 f𝟛
C. 30 f𝟛
D. 50 f𝟛

45 A patient must receive a total of 2.4 g of fenoprofen calcium (Nalfon) P.O. per day, in divided doses. How many milligrams should the patient receive daily?

A. 24 mg
B. 100 mg
C. 2,400 mg
D. 4,600 mg

46 A patient has been given methadone (Dolophine) for several months at a dosage of 0.08 g P.O. daily. This narcotic analgesic is available in 40-mg tablets. How many tablets does the patient receive daily?

A. 1 tablet
B. 2 tablets
C. 10 tablets
D. 20 tablets

47 A patient is to receive gr $\overline{\text{iss}}$ of the hypnotic pentobarbital (Nembutal) P.O. for nighttime sedation. Available capsules are 100 mg each. How many capsules should be administered?

A. ½ capsule
B. ¾ capsule
C. 1 capsule
D. 2 capsules

48 The antibiotic neomycin sulfate (Mycifradin) 1,000 mg P.O. has been ordered. The bottle is labeled 125 mg = 1 ml. How many milliliters must be administered?

A. 8 ml
B. 16 ml
C. 20.5 ml
D. 40 ml

49 A patient is to receive the coronary vasodilator nitroglycerin (Nitrostat). Each tablet equals ⅟₁₅₀ gr. The order is 0.4 mg sublingually. How many tablets must be administered?

A. ½ tablet
B. 1 tablet
C. 2 tablets
D. 2½ tablets

Answer sheet

	A	B	C	D			A	B	C	D
1	○	○	○	○		31	○	○	○	○
2	○	○	○	○		32	○	○	○	○
3	○	○	○	○		33	○	○	○	○
4	○	○	○	○		34	○	○	○	○
5	○	○	○	○		35	○	○	○	○
6	○	○	○	○		36	○	○	○	○
7	○	○	○	○		37	○	○	○	○
8	○	○	○	○		38	○	○	○	○
9	○	○	○	○		39	○	○	○	○
10	○	○	○	○		40	○	○	○	○
11	○	○	○	○		41	○	○	○	○
12	○	○	○	○		42	○	○	○	○
13	○	○	○	○		43	○	○	○	○
14	○	○	○	○		44	○	○	○	○
15	○	○	○	○		45	○	○	○	○
16	○	○	○	○		46	○	○	○	○
17	○	○	○	○		47	○	○	○	○
18	○	○	○	○		48	○	○	○	○
19	○	○	○	○		49	○	○	○	○
20	○	○	○	○						
21	○	○	○	○						
22	○	○	○	○						
23	○	○	○	○						
24	○	○	○	○						
25	○	○	○	○						
26	○	○	○	○						
27	○	○	○	○						
28	○	○	○	○						
29	○	○	○	○						
30	○	○	○	○						

Answers

1 Correct answer — **B**

D/A

$$0.1 \text{ g} \times \frac{1,000 \text{ mg}}{1 \text{ g}} \times \frac{5 \text{ ml}}{125 \text{ mg}} = \frac{500 \text{ ml}}{125} = 4 \text{ ml}$$

R/P

Step 1: Change grams to milligrams.

$$1 \text{ g} : 1,000 \text{ mg} :: 0.1 \text{ g} : x \text{ mg}$$
$$x = 1,000 \times 0.1$$
$$x = 100 \text{ mg}$$

Step 2: Calculate required milliliters.

$$125 \text{ mg} : 5 \text{ ml} :: 100 \text{ mg} : x \text{ ml}$$
$$125x = 5 \times 100$$
$$125x = 500$$
$$x = \frac{500}{125}$$
$$x = 4 \text{ ml}$$

2 Correct answer — **A**

D/A

$$0.25 \text{ mg} \times \frac{1 \text{ ml}}{0.05 \text{ mg}} = \frac{0.25 \text{ ml}}{0.05} = 5 \text{ ml}$$

R/P

$$0.05 \text{ mg} : 1 \text{ ml} :: 0.25 \text{ mg} : x \text{ ml}$$
$$0.05x = 0.25$$
$$x = \frac{0.25}{0.05}$$
$$x = 5 \text{ ml}$$

3 Correct answer — **C**

D/A

$$5 \text{ mg} \times \frac{1 \text{ tab}}{2.5 \text{ mg}} = \frac{5 \text{ tab}}{2.5} = 2 \text{ tablets}$$

R/P

$$2.5 \text{ mg} : 1 \text{ tab} :: 5 \text{ mg} : x \text{ tab}$$
$$2.5x = 5$$
$$x = \frac{5}{2.5}$$
$$x = 2 \text{ tablets}$$

4 Correct answer — **A**

Remember: 1,000 mg = 1 g

D/A

$$1,000 \text{ mg} \times \frac{1 \text{ g}}{1,000 \text{ mg}} \times \frac{1 \text{ tab}}{0.5 \text{ g}} = \frac{1,000 \text{ tab}}{500} = 2 \text{ tablets}$$

R/P

$$0.5 \text{ g} : 1 \text{ tab} :: 1 \text{ g} : x \text{ tab}$$
$$0.5x = 1$$
$$x = \frac{1}{0.5}$$
$$x = 2 \text{ tablets}$$

5 Correct answer — **D**

D/A

$$300 \text{ mg} \times \frac{5 \text{ ml}}{100 \text{ mg}} = \frac{1,500}{100} = 15 \text{ ml}$$

R/P

$$100 \text{ mg} : 5 \text{ ml} :: 300 \text{ mg} : x \text{ ml}$$
$$100x = 5 \times 300$$
$$100x = 1,500$$
$$x = \frac{1,500}{100}$$
$$x = 15 \text{ ml}$$

6 Correct answer — **C**

D/A

$$1.5 \text{ g} \times \frac{1,000 \text{ mg}}{1 \text{ g}} \times \frac{1 \text{ tab}}{500 \text{ mg}} = \frac{1,500 \text{ tab}}{500} = 3 \text{ tablets}$$

R/P

Step 1: Change grams to milligrams.
$$1 \text{ g} : 1,000 \text{ mg} :: 1.5 \text{ g} : x \text{ mg}$$
$$x = 1,000 \times 1.5$$
$$x = 1,500 \text{ mg}$$

Step 2: Calculate required tablets.
$$500 \text{ mg} : 1 \text{ tab} :: 1,500 \text{ mg} : x \text{ tab}$$
$$500x = 1,500$$
$$x = \frac{1,500}{500}$$
$$x = 3 \text{ tablets}$$

7 Correct answer—**B**

D/A

$$0.25 \text{ mg} \times \frac{1 \text{ tab}}{0.125 \text{ mg}} = \frac{0.25 \text{ tab}}{0.125} = 2 \text{ tablets}$$

R/P

$$0.125 \text{ mg} : 1 \text{ tab} :: 0.25 \text{ mg} : x \text{ tab}$$
$$0.125x = 0.25$$
$$x = \frac{0.25}{0.125}$$
$$x = 2 \text{ tablets}$$

8 Correct answer—**A**

D/A

$$50 \text{ mg} \times \frac{1 \text{ tab}}{12.5 \text{ mg}} = \frac{50 \text{ tab}}{12.5} = 4 \text{ tablets}$$

R/P

$$12.5 \text{ mg} : 1 \text{ tab} :: 50 \text{ mg} : x \text{ tab}$$
$$12.5x = 50$$
$$x = \frac{50}{12.5}$$
$$x = 4 \text{ tablets}$$

9 Correct answer—**A**

D/A

$$300 \text{ mg} \times \frac{5 \text{ ml}}{500 \text{ mg}} = \frac{1,500 \text{ ml}}{500} = 3 \text{ ml}$$

R/P

$$500 \text{ mg} : 5 \text{ ml} :: 300 \text{ mg} : x \text{ ml}$$
$$500x = 1,500$$
$$x = \frac{1,500}{500}$$
$$x = 3 \text{ ml}$$

10 Correct answer—**A**

D/A

$$400,000 \text{ U} \times \frac{5 \text{ ml}}{500,000 \text{ U}} = \frac{20 \text{ ml}}{5} = 4 \text{ ml}$$

R/P

$$500,000 \text{ U} : 5 \text{ ml} :: 400,000 \text{ U} : x \text{ ml}$$
$$500,000x = 5 \times 400,000$$
$$500,000x = 2,000,000$$
$$x = \frac{2,000,000}{500,000}$$
$$x = 4 \text{ ml}$$

11

Correct answer — **B**

Remember: A 50% solution = 50 g per 100 ml.

D/A

$$25 \ \cancel{g} \times \frac{100 \text{ ml}}{50 \ \cancel{g}} = \frac{2,500 \text{ ml}}{50} = 50 \text{ ml}$$

R/P

$$50 \text{ g} : 100 \text{ ml} :: 25 \text{ g} : x \text{ ml}$$
$$50x = 100 \times 25$$
$$50x = 2,500$$
$$x = \frac{2,500}{50}$$
$$x = 50 \text{ ml}$$

12

Correct answer — **C**

D/A

$$0.8 \ \cancel{g} \times \frac{1,000 \ \cancel{mg}}{1 \ \cancel{g}} \times \frac{1 \text{ tab}}{400 \ \cancel{mg}} = \frac{800 \text{ tab}}{400} = 2 \text{ tablets}$$

R/P

Step 1: Change grams to milligrams.

$$1 \text{ g} : 1,000 \text{ mg} :: 0.8 \text{ g} : x \text{ mg}$$
$$x = 1,000 \times 0.8$$
$$x = 800 \text{ mg}$$

Step 2: Calculate required tablets.

$$400 \text{ mg} : 1 \text{ tab} :: 800 \text{ mg} : x \text{ tab}$$
$$400x = 800$$
$$x = \frac{800}{400}$$
$$x = 2 \text{ tablets}$$

13

Correct answer — **D**

D/A

$$12 \ \cancel{mg} \times \frac{1 \text{ tab}}{2 \ \cancel{mg}} = \frac{12 \text{ tab}}{2} = 6 \text{ tablets}$$

R/P

$$2 \text{ mg} : 1 \text{ tab} :: 12 \text{ mg} : x \text{ tab}$$
$$2x = 12$$
$$x = \frac{12}{2}$$
$$x = 6 \text{ tablets}$$

---

14 Correct answer—**C**

Remember: 1 gr = 60 mg

D/A

$$3 \text{ gr} \times \frac{60 \text{ mg}}{1 \text{ gr}} \times \frac{1 \text{ tab}}{100 \text{ mg}} = \frac{180 \text{ tab}}{100} = 1\tfrac{4}{5} \text{ or } 2 \text{ tablets}$$

R/P

$$100 \text{ mg} : 1 \text{ tab} :: 180 \text{ mg} : x \text{ tab}$$
$$100x = 180$$
$$x = \frac{180}{100}$$
$$x = 1\tfrac{4}{5} \text{ or } 2 \text{ tablets}$$

---

15 Correct answer—**A**

D/A

$$1.2 \text{ mg} \times \frac{1,000 \text{ mcg}}{1 \text{ mg}} \times \frac{1 \text{ tab}}{600 \text{ mcg}} = \frac{1,200 \text{ tab}}{600} = 2 \text{ tablets}$$

R/P

Step 1: Change milligrams to micrograms.
$$1 \text{ mg} : 1,000 \text{ mcg} :: 1.2 \text{ mg} : x \text{ mcg}$$
$$x = 1,000 \times 1.2$$
$$x = 1,200 \text{ mcg}$$

Step 2: Calculate required tablets.
$$600 \text{ mcg} : 1 \text{ tab} :: 1,200 \text{ mcg} : x \text{ tab}$$
$$600x = 1,200$$
$$x = \frac{1,200}{600}$$
$$x = 2 \text{ tablets}$$

---

16 Correct answer—**B**

D/A

$$2,000 \text{ mg} \times \frac{1 \text{ tab}}{500 \text{ mg}} = \frac{20 \text{ tab}}{5} = 4 \text{ tablets}$$

R/P

$$500 \text{ mg} : 1 \text{ tab} :: 2{,}000 \text{ mg} : x \text{ tab}$$
$$500x = 2{,}000$$
$$x = \frac{2{,}000}{500}$$
$$x = 4 \text{ tablets}$$

17 Correct answer — **D**

D/A

$$\frac{1}{6} \cancel{\text{gr}} \times \frac{60 \cancel{\text{mg}}}{1 \cancel{\text{gr}}} \times \frac{1 \text{ tab}}{5 \cancel{\text{mg}}} = \frac{60 \text{ tab}}{30} = 2 \text{ tablets}$$

R/P

Step 1: Change grains to milligrams.
$$1 \text{ gr} : 60 \text{ mg} :: \tfrac{1}{6} \text{ gr} : x \text{ mg}$$
$$x = 60 \times \tfrac{1}{6}$$
$$x = 10 \text{ mg}$$

Step 2: Calculate required tablets.
$$5 \text{ mg} : 1 \text{ tab} :: 10 \text{ mg} : x \text{ tab}$$
$$5x = 10$$
$$x = \frac{10}{5}$$
$$x = 2 \text{ tablets}$$

18 Correct answer — **C**

D/A

$$0.25 \cancel{\text{mg}} \times \frac{1{,}000 \cancel{\text{mcg}}}{1 \cancel{\text{mg}}} \times \frac{1 \text{ ml}}{50 \cancel{\text{mcg}}} = \frac{250 \text{ ml}}{50} = 5 \text{ ml}$$

R/P

Step 1: Change milligrams to micrograms.
$$1 \text{ mg} : 1{,}000 \text{ mcg} :: 0.25 \text{ mg} : x \text{ mcg}$$
$$x = 1{,}000 \times 0.25$$
$$x = 250 \text{ mcg}$$

Step 2: Calculate required milliliters.
$$50 \text{ mcg} : 1 \text{ ml} :: 250 \text{ mcg} : x \text{ ml}$$
$$50x = 250$$
$$x = \frac{250}{50}$$
$$x = 5 \text{ ml}$$

19 Correct answer — **C**

D/A

$$5 \text{ gtt} \times \frac{1 \text{ ml}}{15 \text{ gtt}} = \frac{5 \text{ ml}}{15} = 0.3 \text{ ml}$$

R/P

$$15 \text{ gtt} : 1 \text{ ml} :: 5 \text{ gtt} : x \text{ ml}$$
$$15x = 5$$
$$x = \frac{5}{15}$$
$$x = 0.3 \text{ ml}$$

20 Correct answer — **A**

D/A

$$0.2 \text{ ml} \times \frac{15 \text{ gtt}}{1 \text{ ml}} = 3 \text{ gtt}$$

R/P

$$1 \text{ ml} : 15 \text{ gtt} :: 0.2 \text{ ml} : x \text{ gtt}$$
$$x = 15 \times 0.2$$
$$x = 3 \text{ gtt}$$

21 Correct answer — **A**

Remember: gtt = ℞. This is an equivalent.

D/A

$$8 \text{ gtt} = 8 \text{ ℞}$$

R/P

$$8 \text{ gtt} = 8 \text{ ℞}$$

22 Correct answer — **C**

D/A

$$0.1 \text{ g} \times \frac{1,000 \text{ mg}}{1 \text{ g}} \times \frac{1 \text{ tab}}{50 \text{ mg}} = \frac{100 \text{ tab}}{50} = 2 \text{ tablets}$$

R/P

Step 1: Change grams to milligrams.
$$1 \text{ g} : 1,000 \text{ mg} :: 0.1 \text{ g} : x \text{ mg}$$
$$x = 1,000 \times 0.1$$
$$x = 100 \text{ mg}$$

Step 2: Calculate required tablets.
$$50 \text{ mg} : 1 \text{ tab} :: 100 \text{ mg} : x \text{ tab}$$
$$50x = 100$$
$$x = \frac{100}{50}$$
$$x = 2 \text{ tablets}$$

23 Correct answer—**D**

D/A

$$1.5 \not{g} \times \frac{1,000 \not{mg}}{1 \not{g}} \times \frac{1 \text{ tab}}{500 \not{mg}} = \frac{1,500 \text{ tab}}{500} = 3 \text{ tablets}$$

R/P

Step 1: Change grams to milligrams.

$$1 \text{ g} : 1,000 \text{ mg} :: 1.5 \text{ g} : x \text{ mg}$$
$$x = 1,000 \times 1.5$$
$$x = 1,500 \text{ mg}$$

Step 2: Calculate required tablets.

$$500 \text{ mg} : 1 \text{ tab} :: 1,500 \text{ mg} : x \text{ tab}$$
$$500x = 1,500$$
$$x = \frac{1,500}{500}$$
$$x = 3 \text{ tablets}$$

24 Correct answer—**C**

D/A

$$1.2 \not{mg} \times \frac{1 \text{ tab}}{0.3 \not{mg}} = \frac{1.2 \text{ tab}}{0.3} = 4 \text{ tablets}$$

R/P

$$0.3 \text{ mg} : 1 \text{ tab} :: 1.2 \text{ mg} : x \text{ tab}$$
$$0.3x = 1.2$$
$$x = \frac{1.2}{0.3}$$
$$x = 4 \text{ tablets}$$

25 Correct answer—**D**

D/A

$$10 \not{mg} \times \frac{1 \text{ tab}}{2.5 \not{mg}} = \frac{10 \text{ tab}}{2.5} = 4 \text{ tablets}$$

R/P

$$2.5 \text{ mg} : 1 \text{ tab} :: 10 \text{ mg} : x \text{ tab}$$
$$2.5x = 10$$
$$x = \frac{10}{2.5}$$
$$x = 4 \text{ tablets}$$

26 Correct answer — **D**

D/A

$$1.2\ \cancel{g} \times \frac{1,000\ \cancel{mg}}{1\ \cancel{g}} \times \frac{1\ cap}{300\ \cancel{mg}} = \frac{1,200\ cap}{300} = 4\ capsules$$

R/P

Step 1: Change grams to milligrams.

$$1\ g : 1,000\ mg :: 1.2\ g : x\ mg$$
$$x = 1,000 \times 1.2$$
$$x = 1,200\ mg$$

Step 2: Calculate required capsules.

$$300\ mg : 1\ cap :: 1,200\ mg : x\ cap$$
$$300x = 1,200$$
$$x = \frac{1,200}{300}$$
$$x = 4\ capsules$$

27 Correct answer — **C**

D/A

$$8\ \cancel{mg} \times \frac{0.5\ ml}{0.5\ \cancel{mg}} = 8\ ml$$

R/P

$$0.5\ mg : 0.5\ ml :: 8\ mg : x\ ml$$
$$0.5x = 0.5 \times 8$$
$$0.5x = 4$$
$$x = \frac{4}{0.5}$$
$$x = 8\ ml$$

28 Correct answer — **A**

D/A

$$50\ \cancel{mg} \times \frac{4\ ml}{12.5\ \cancel{mg}} = \frac{200\ ml}{12.5} = 16\ ml$$

R/P

$$12.5\ mg : 4\ ml :: 50\ mg : x\ ml$$
$$12.5x = 200$$
$$x = \frac{200}{12.5}$$
$$x = 16\ ml$$

29 Correct answer—**D**

D/A

$$1 \text{ mg} \times \frac{1 \text{ cap}}{0.25 \text{ mg}} = \frac{1 \text{ cap}}{0.25} = 4 \text{ capsules}$$

R/P

$$0.25 \text{ mg} : 1 \text{ cap} :: 1 \text{ mg} : x \text{ cap}$$
$$0.25x = 1$$
$$x = \frac{1}{0.25}$$
$$x = 4 \text{ capsules}$$

30 Correct answer—**B**

D/A

$$0.1 \text{ mg} \times \frac{1,000 \text{ mcg}}{1 \text{ mg}} \times \frac{1 \text{ tab}}{50 \text{ mcg}} = \frac{100 \text{ tab}}{50} = 2 \text{ tablets}$$

R/P

Step 1: Change milligrams to micrograms.
$$1 \text{ mg} : 1,000 \text{ mcg} :: 0.1 \text{ mg} : x \text{ mcg}$$
$$x = 1,000 \times 0.1$$
$$x = 100 \text{ mcg}$$

Step 2: Calculate required tablets.
$$50 \text{ mcg} : 1 \text{ tab} :: 100 \text{ mcg} : x \text{ tab}$$
$$50x = 100$$
$$x = \frac{100}{50}$$
$$x = 2 \text{ tablets}$$

31 Correct answer—**B**

D/A

$$1.3 \text{ g} \times \frac{1,000 \text{ mg}}{1 \text{ g}} \times \frac{1 \text{ tab}}{325 \text{ mg}} = \frac{1,300 \text{ tab}}{325} = 4 \text{ tablets}$$

R/P

Step 1: Change grams to milligrams.
$$1 \text{ g} : 1,000 \text{ mg} :: 1.3 \text{ g} : x \text{ mg}$$
$$x = 1,000 \times 1.3$$
$$x = 1,300 \text{ mg}$$

Step 2: Calculate required tablets.

$$325 \text{ mg} : 1 \text{ tab} :: 1{,}300 \text{ mg} : x \text{ tab}$$
$$325x = 1{,}300$$
$$x = \frac{1{,}300}{325}$$
$$x = 4 \text{ tablets}$$

32 Correct answer – C

D/A

$$1{,}\cancel{000{,}000}\ \cancel{U} \times \frac{5 \text{ ml}}{2\cancel{00{,}000}\ \cancel{U}} = \frac{50 \text{ ml}}{2} = 25 \text{ ml}$$

R/P

$$200{,}000 \text{ U} : 5 \text{ ml} :: 1{,}000{,}000 \text{ U} : x \text{ ml}$$
$$200{,}000x = 5{,}000{,}000 \text{ U}$$
$$x = \frac{5{,}000{,}000}{200{,}000}$$
$$x = 25 \text{ ml}$$

33 Correct answer – A

D/A

$$6\cancel{00{,}000}\ \cancel{U} \times \frac{1 \text{ ml}}{1\cancel{00{,}000}\ \cancel{U}} = 6 \text{ ml}$$

R/P

$$100{,}000 \text{ U} : 1 \text{ ml} :: 600{,}000 \text{ U} : x \text{ ml}$$
$$100{,}000x = 600{,}000$$
$$x = \frac{600{,}000}{100{,}000}$$
$$x = 6 \text{ ml}$$

34 Correct answer – D

D/A

$$2\ \cancel{f\mathfrak{z}} \times \frac{30 \text{ ml}}{1\ \cancel{f\mathfrak{z}}} = 60 \text{ ml}$$

R/P

$$1\ f\mathfrak{z} : 30 \text{ ml} :: 2\ f\mathfrak{z} : x \text{ ml}$$
$$x = 30 \times 2$$
$$x = 60 \text{ ml}$$

35 Correct answer—**B**

Remember: 5 ml = 1 tsp

D/A

$$5 \text{ ml} \times \frac{1 \text{ tsp}}{5 \text{ ml}} = 1 \text{ tsp}$$

R/P

$$5 \text{ ml} : 1 \text{ tsp} :: 5 \text{ ml} : x \text{ tsp}$$
$$5x = 5$$
$$x = \frac{5}{5}$$
$$x = 1 \text{ tsp}$$

36 Correct answer—**D**

D/A

$$400 \text{ calories} \times \frac{1 \text{ g}}{3.8 \text{ calories}} = \frac{400 \text{ g}}{3.8} = 105.3 \text{ or } 105 \text{ g}$$

R/P

$$3.8 \text{ calories} : 1 \text{ g} :: 400 \text{ calories} : x \text{ g}$$
$$3.8x = 400$$
$$x = \frac{400}{3.8}$$
$$x = 105.3 \text{ or } 105 \text{ g}$$

37 Correct answer—**A**

D/A

$$80 \text{ calories} \times \frac{1 \text{ ml}}{1.5 \text{ calories}} = \frac{80 \text{ ml}}{1.5} = 53.3 \text{ or } 53 \text{ ml}$$

R/P

$$1.5 \text{ calories} : 1 \text{ ml} :: 80 \text{ calories} : x \text{ ml}$$
$$1.5x = 80$$
$$x = \frac{80}{1.5}$$
$$x = 53.3 \text{ ml or } 53 \text{ ml}$$

38 Correct answer—**B**

D/A

$$0.3\ \cancel{g} \times \frac{1{,}000\ \cancel{mg}}{1\ \cancel{g}} \times \frac{1\ tab}{50\ \cancel{mg}} = \frac{300\ tab}{50} = 6\ tablets$$

R/P

Step 1: Change grams to milligrams.

$$1\ g : 1{,}000\ mg :: 0.3\ g : x\ mg$$
$$x = 1{,}000 \times 0.3$$
$$x = 300\ mg$$

Step 2: Calculate required tablets.

$$50\ mg : 1\ tab :: 300\ mg : x\ tab$$
$$50x = 300$$
$$x = \frac{300}{50}$$
$$x = 6\ tablets$$

39 Correct answer—**D**

D/A

$$225\ \cancel{mg} \times \frac{1\ tab}{75\ \cancel{mg}} = \frac{225\ tab}{75} = 3\ tablets$$

R/P

$$75\ mg : 1\ tab :: 225\ mg : x\ tab$$
$$75x = 225$$
$$x = \frac{225}{75}$$
$$x = 3\ tablets$$

40 Correct answer—**D**

D/A

$$0.5\ \cancel{g} \times \frac{1{,}000\ \cancel{mg}}{1\ \cancel{g}} \times \frac{1\ ml}{62.5\ \cancel{mg}} = \frac{500\ ml}{62.5} = 8\ ml$$

R/P

Step 1: Change grams to milligrams.

$$1\ g : 1{,}000\ mg :: 0.5\ g : x\ mg$$
$$x = 1{,}000 \times 0.5$$
$$x = 500\ mg$$

Step 2: Calculate required milliliters.

$$62.5\ mg : 1\ ml :: 500\ mg : x\ ml$$
$$62.5x = 500$$
$$x = \frac{500}{62.5}$$
$$x = 8\ ml$$

41 Correct answer — **A**

D/A

$$0.4\ \cancel{g} \times \frac{1{,}000\ \cancel{mg}}{1\ \cancel{g}} \times \frac{1\ \text{tab}}{100\ \cancel{mg}} = \frac{400\ \text{tab}}{100} = 4\ \text{tablets}$$

R/P

Step 1: Change grams to milligrams.

$$1\ g : 1{,}000\ mg :: 0.4\ g : x\ \text{tab}$$
$$x = 1{,}000 \times 0.4$$
$$x = 400\ mg$$

Step 2: Calculate required tablets.

$$100\ mg : 1\ \text{tab} :: 400\ mg : x\ \text{tab}$$
$$100x = 400$$
$$x = \frac{400}{100}$$
$$x = 4\ \text{tablets}$$

42 Correct answer — **D**

D/A

$$30\ \cancel{g} \times \frac{15\ ml}{10\ \cancel{g}} = \frac{450\ ml}{10} = 45\ ml$$

R/P

$$10\ g : 15\ ml :: 30\ g : x\ ml$$
$$10x = 15 \times 30$$
$$10x = 450$$
$$x = \frac{450}{10}$$
$$x = 45\ ml$$

43 Correct answer — **C**

Remember: 1 g = 1,000 mg

D/A

$$1\ \cancel{g} \times \frac{1{,}000\ \cancel{mg}}{1\ \cancel{g}} \times \frac{1\ \text{tab}}{250\ \cancel{mg}} = \frac{1{,}000\ \text{tab}}{250} = 4\ \text{tablets}$$

R/P

$$250\ mg : 1\ \text{tab} :: 1{,}000\ mg : x\ \text{tab}$$
$$250x = 1{,}000$$
$$x = \frac{1{,}000}{250}$$
$$x = 4\ \text{tablets}$$

44 Correct answer — **A**

D/A

$$200 \text{ mg} \times \frac{5 \text{ ml}}{50 \text{ mg}} \times \frac{1 \text{ f}ʒ}{5 \text{ ml}} = \frac{200 \text{ f}ʒ}{50} = 4 \text{ f}ʒ$$

R/P

Step 1: Calculate required milliliters.

$$50 \text{ mg} : 5 \text{ ml} :: 200 \text{ mg} : x \text{ ml}$$
$$50x = 5 \times 200$$
$$50x = 1,000$$
$$x = \frac{1,000}{50}$$
$$x = 20 \text{ ml}$$

Step 2: Change milliliters to fluidrams.

$$5 \text{ ml} : 1 \text{ f}ʒ :: 20 \text{ ml} : x \text{ f}ʒ$$
$$5x = 20$$
$$x = \frac{20}{5}$$
$$x = 4 \text{ f}ʒ$$

45 Correct answer — **C**

D/A

$$2.4 \text{ g} \times \frac{1,000 \text{ mg}}{1 \text{ g}} = 2,400 \text{ mg}$$

R/P

$$1 \text{ g} : 1,000 \text{ mg} :: 2.4 \text{ g} : x \text{ mg}$$
$$x = 1,000 \times 2.4$$
$$x = 2,400 \text{ mg}$$

46 Correct answer — **B**

D/A

$$0.08 \text{ g} \times \frac{1,000 \text{ mg}}{1 \text{ g}} \times \frac{1 \text{ tab}}{40 \text{ mg}} = \frac{80 \text{ tab}}{40} = 2 \text{ tablets}$$

R/P

Step 1: Change grams to milligrams.

$$1 \text{ g} : 1,000 \text{ mg} :: 0.08 \text{ g} : x \text{ mg}$$
$$x = 1,000 \times 0.08$$
$$x = 80 \text{ mg}$$

Step 2: Calculate required tablets.

$$40 \text{ mg} : 1 \text{ tab} :: 80 \text{ mg} : x \text{ tab}$$
$$40x = 80$$
$$x = \frac{80}{40}$$
$$x = 2 \text{ tablets}$$

47 Correct answer—C

D/A

$$\tfrac{3}{2}\ \text{gr} \times \frac{60\ \text{mg}}{1\ \text{gr}} \times \frac{1\ \text{cap}}{100\ \text{mg}} = \frac{180\ \text{cap}}{200} = \frac{9\ \text{cap}}{10} = 1\ \text{capsule}$$

R/P

Step 1: Change grains to milligrams.

$$1\ \text{gr} : 60\ \text{mg} :: 1\tfrac{1}{2}\ \text{gr} : x\ \text{mg}$$
$$x = 60 \times 1.5$$
$$x = 90\ \text{mg}$$

Step 2: Calculate required capsules.

$$100\ \text{mg} : 1\ \text{cap} :: 90\ \text{mg} : x\ \text{cap}$$
$$100x = 90$$
$$x = \frac{90}{100}$$
$$x = \tfrac{9}{10}\ \text{or}\ 1\ \text{capsule}$$

48 Correct answer—A

D/A

$$1{,}000\ \text{mg} \times \frac{1\ \text{ml}}{125\ \text{mg}} = \frac{1{,}000\ \text{ml}}{125} = 8\ \text{ml}$$

R/P

$$125\ \text{mg} : 1\ \text{ml} :: 1{,}000\ \text{mg} : x\ \text{ml}$$
$$125x = 1{,}000$$
$$x = \frac{1{,}000}{125}$$
$$x = 8\ \text{ml}$$

49 Correct answer—B

D/A

$$0.4\ \text{mg} \times \frac{1\ \text{gr}}{60\ \text{mg}} \times \frac{1\ \text{tab}}{\tfrac{1}{150}\ \text{gr}} = \frac{0.4\ \text{tab}}{\tfrac{60}{150}} = \frac{0.4\ \text{tab}}{0.4} = 1\ \text{tablet}$$

R/P

$$60\ \text{mg} : 1\ \text{gr} :: 0.4\ \text{mg} : x\ \text{gr}$$
$$60x = 0.4$$
$$x = \frac{0.4}{60} = \tfrac{4}{600}$$
$$x = \tfrac{1}{150}\ \text{gr}$$

Because each tablet contains $\tfrac{1}{150}$ gr, give 1 tablet.

CHAPTER 5

Parenteral Medications

Questions

1 The physician has ordered $\frac{1}{300}$ gr I.M. of the anticholinergic drug atropine. The label reads 1 ml = $\frac{1}{150}$ gr. What is the equivalent dose in milliliters?

A. 0.08 ml
B. 0.125 ml
C. 0.5 ml
D. 1.25 ml

2 The physician's order reads "Administer 500 mg of methicillin (Staphcillin) I.M." The vial is labeled 6 g = 6 ml. How many milliliters of this antibiotic should the nurse administer?

A. 0.5 ml
B. 1 ml
C. 1.6 ml
D. 2.4 ml

3 The physician orders digoxin (Lanoxin) 0.125 mg I.M. The ampule reads 1 ml = 0.25 mg. How many milliliters of this cardiac glycoside should be prepared?

A. 0.25 ml
B. 0.5 ml
C. 0.75 ml
D. 1 ml

4 A vial of dacarbazine (DTIC-Dome), an antineoplastic drug, is labeled 100 mg = 10 ml. How many milliliters should be prepared for a patient weighing 50 kg if the order were for 2 mg/kg I.V.?

A. 2 ml
B. 10 ml
C. 25 ml
D. 50 ml

5 A vial of dactinomycin (actinomycin D, Cosmegen) reads 0.5 mg = 1 ml. A patient weighing 60 kg is to receive 15 mcg/kg I.M. How many milliliters of this antibiotic antineoplastic drug should be prepared?

A. 0.125 ml
B. 0.6 ml
C. 0.8 ml
D. 1.8 ml

6 The physician has ordered salmon calcitonin (Calcimar) 100 IU I.M. to lower a patient's extracellular fluid calcium level. The vial label reads 200 IU/ml. How many milliliters of this hormone should be administered?

A. 0.5 ml
B. 1.5 ml
C. 2.6 ml
D. 7 ml

7 The physician orders cefoxitin (Mefoxin) 500 mg I.M. q12h. The vial label reads 1 ml = 400 mg. How many milliliters of this antibiotic should be given every 12 hours?

A. 0.025 ml
B. 0.125 ml
C. 1.25 ml
D. 12.5 ml

8 A patient must receive 0.25 g I.M. of cefazolin (Ancef), an antibiotic. The label reads 125 mg = 1 ml. How many milliliters should be administered?

A. 0.1 ml
B. 1 ml
C. 2 ml
D. 10 ml

9 The nurse must prepare 40 mEq of the electrolyte potassium chloride (Kaon-Cl) from a vial labeled 2 mEq = 1 ml. How many milliliters equal 40 mEq?

A. 15 ml
B. 20 ml
C. 32 ml
D. 125 ml

10 The physician orders 1,200,000 U of penicillin G potassium (Lanacillin) I.M. The vial is labeled 10 ml = 6,000,000 U. How many milliliters equal the prescribed dose?

A. 0.06 ml
B. 0.18 ml
C. 1 ml
D. 2 ml

11 The physician's order reads "Administer 0.02 g furosemide (Lasix) I.M." The vial is labeled 20 mg = 1 ml. How many milliliters of this diuretic equal 0.02 g?

A. 1 ml
B. 20 ml
C. 100 ml
D. 250 ml

12 The physician has ordered 100 mg of the mineral calcium gluceptate I.V. The vial is labeled 5 ml = 1.1 g. How many milliliters should be administered?

A. 0.015 ml
B. 0.08 ml
C. 0.45 ml
D. 32 ml

13 What amount of the narcotic codeine phosphate should be withdrawn from a vial labeled 1 ml = 15 mg if the prescription reads "gr s̄s̄ I.M."?

A. 0.6 ml
B. 1 ml
C. 1.7 ml
D. 2 ml

14 The physician orders 7,500 U of the parenteral anticoagulant heparin S.C. daily; the ampule reads 1 ml = 5,000 U. How many milliliters should be administered?

A. 0.6 ml
B. 1.2 ml
C. 1.5 ml
D. 2 ml

15 If the above order were changed to 2,500 U heparin S.C. daily, how many minims would be administered?

A. 3 ℥
B. 4.5 ℥
C. 7.5 ℥
D. 10 ℥

16 A patient must receive 0.2 g of isoniazid (Nydrazid), an antitubercular drug, by intramuscular injection. The vial is labeled 100 mg = 1 ml. How many milliliters should be administered?

A. 0.2 ml
B. 0.4 ml
C. 1.2 ml
D. 2 ml

17 The physician orders 0.5 g I.V. of the bronchodilator aminophylline (Somophyllin). The ampule reads 10 ml = 10 g. How many milliliters equal 0.5 g?

A. 0.25 ml
B. 0.5 ml
C. 1.25 ml
D. 15 ml

18 A patient is to receive 60 U of isophane insulin suspension (NPH) S.C. daily. The vial is labeled 100 U = 1 ml. How many milliliters of this pancreatic hormone must be administered?

A. 0.09 ml
B. 0.2 ml
C. 0.6 ml
D. 45 ml

19 The physician's order reads "Atropine sulfate $\frac{1}{100}$ gr I.M." If the vial is labeled $\frac{1}{150}$ gr = 1 ml, how many milliliters of this anticholinergic drug should the nurse administer?

A. 0.33 ml
B. 0.5 ml
C. 1 ml
D. 1.5 ml

20 The physician orders 0.25 g of the antibiotic streptomycin sulfate I.M. The vial reads 2 ml = 1 g. How many milliliters should be administered?

A. 0.1 ml
B. 0.25 ml
C. 0.5 ml
D. 3 ml

21 The physician orders 5 mg of the narcotic morphine sulfate S.C. stat. The vial reads 1 ml = 1/10 gr. How many minims should be administered?

A. 4 ♏
B. 13 ♏
C. 28 ♏
D. 70 ♏

22 How many milliliters of the preparation iron dextran (Imferon) should be administered if the physician's order is 0.1 g I.M. and the label reads 50 mg = 1 ml?

A. 1 ml
B. 2 ml
C. 2.5 ml
D. 4 ml

23 The physician orders 0.1 g I.V. push of procainamide (Pronestyl), an antiarrhythmic preparation. The vial is labeled 100 mg = 1 ml. How many milliliters must be administered?

A. 0.1 ml
B. 1 ml
C. 28 ml
D. 48 ml

24 A patient with a body-surface area (BSA) of 1.5 m^2 is to receive the antineoplastic drug mechlorethamine (nitrogen mustard, Mustargen) 6 mg/m^2 as a single intravenous dose. The vial is labeled 1 ml = 10 mg. How many milliliters should be prepared?

A. 0.25 ml
B. 0.45 ml
C. 0.9 ml
D. 1.8 ml

25 The physician orders 0.5 mg of epinephrine (Epitrate) 1:10,000 I.M. The 10-ml ampule is labeled 0.1 mg/ml (1:10,000). How many milliliters of this sympathomimetic drug should be given?

A. 5 ml
B. 15 ml
C. 80 ml
D. 126 ml

26 A patient is to receive the narcotic antagonist naloxone hydrochloride (Narcan), 1.2 mg intravenously. The ampule is labeled 0.4 mg/ml. How many milliliters must be prepared?

A. 0.12 ml
B. 0.45 ml
C. 3 ml
D. 12.5 ml

27 Scopolamine hydrobromide ½₀₀ gr I.M. has been ordered because of its antimuscarinic (anticholinergic) properties. The ampule is labeled 0.3 mg = 1 ml. How many milliliters should be given?

A. 0.05 ml
B. 1 ml
C. 1.5 ml
D. 3 ml

28 A patient is to receive 5 U of posterior pituitary hormone (Pituitrin) I.M. If the vial is labeled 10 U/ml, how many milliliters should be administered?

A. 0.038 ml
B. 0.27 ml
C. 0.5 ml
D. 1.25 ml

29 Intravenous therapy with vincristine (Oncovin) has been ordered for a patient because of its antineoplastic properties. The order reads 1.4 mg/m², and the patient's BSA is 1.3 m². The vial is labeled 1 mg = 0.5 ml. How many milliliters should be prepared?

A. 0.3 ml
B. 0.45 ml
C. 0.8 ml
D. 0.9 ml

30 A patient with a BSA of 1.7 m² is to receive a dose of medication at 100 U/m². The vial is labeled 1 ml = 200 U. How many minims should be prepared?

A. 10 ℔
B. 13 ℔
C. 35 ℔
D. 60 ℔

31 A patient who weighs 60 kg is to receive 0.5 mg/kg of a medication. The vial is labeled 1 mg = 1 ℳ. How many milliliters should be administered?

A. 0.3 ml
B. 0.4 ml
C. 0.9 ml
D. 2 ml

32 How many milliliters of the anticonvulsant phenobarbital (Luminal) should be administered to a 45-kg patient if the order reads 10 mg/kg I.V. and the ampule is labeled 1 ml = 130 mg?

A. 0.4 ml
B. 0.8 ml
C. 1 ml
D. 3.5 ml

33 A patient who weighs 50 kg is to receive the sedative midazolam (Versed), 0.07 mg/kg I.M. 30 minutes before surgery. The vial is labeled 1 ml = 5 mg. How many minims should be administered?

A. 7 ℳ
B. 9 ℳ
C. 11 ℳ
D. 18 ℳ

34 Methylprednisolone powder (A-Metha-pred) has the following manufacturer's instructions: "Add 8 ml of bacteriostatic water for injection to vial of 500 mg; then 125 mg/2 ml." How many milliliters of this glucocorticoid are needed for a dose of 50 mg?

A. 0.5 ml
B. 0.8 ml
C. 1 ml
D. 2.4 ml

35 A patient has been placed on antibiotic therapy with ampicillin sodium (Polycillin-N) 0.4 g I.M. q6h. The vial of powder states: "Add 3.5 ml of diluent, and the resulting solution contains 250 mg/ml." How many milliliters of this prepared solution should the patient receive every 6 hours?

A. 1.6 ml
B. 2.3 ml
C. 2.5 ml
D. 3.2 ml

36 The physician orders 500 mg I.M. of cefazolin sulfate (Ancef). The pharmacy supplies a vial of powder with the following instructions: "Add 2.5 ml of sterile water for injection. This will provide an approximate volume of 330 mg/ml." How many milliliters of this antibiotic preparation should be administered?

A. 0.125 ml
B. 0.9 ml
C. 1.5 ml
D. 2.6 ml

37 An I.V. solution of penicillin G potassium, 10,000 U/kg, has been ordered for a patient weighing 55 kg. The available vial, labeled 1,000,000 U and needing reconstitution, is accompanied by these instructions: "Add 19.6 ml of diluent for 50,000 U/ml of solution." How many milliliters of this antibiotic solution must be prepared?

A. 0.2 ml
B. 2 ml
C. 4.5 ml
D. 11 ml

38 How many grams of pure drug are used in preparing 250 ml of a 0.5% solution?

A. 1.25 g
B. 12 g
C. 13.5 g
D. 25 g

39 If 5 g of pure drug have been dissolved in a solution that now measures 250 ml, what percent strength has been made?

A. 2%
B. 4%
C. 10%
D. 20%

40 How many grams of sodium chloride are in 2,000 ml of 0.9% normal saline solution?

A. 2 g
B. 10 g
C. 15 g
D. 18 g

41 How many milliliters of the antiseizure drug magnesium sulfate should be administered from a vial labeled 50% (10 ml) if the order is for 500 mg?

A. 1 ml
B. 2 ml
C. 4 ml
D. 8 ml

42 How many grams of pure drug are in 50 ml of a 25% glucose solution?

A. 3 g
B. 8.75 g
C. 12.5 g
D. 18 g

43 The nurse must prepare a dilute solution of an oral antiseptic, cetylpyridinium chloride (Cepacol), from full-strength cetylpyridinium. How many milliliters of this antiseptic are needed to make 120 ml of the 25% solution?

A. 3 ml
B. 12 ml
C. 30 ml
D. 100 ml

Answer sheet

	A	B	C	D			A	B	C	D
1	○	○	○	○		31	○	○	○	○
2	○	○	○	○		32	○	○	○	○
3	○	○	○	○		33	○	○	○	○
4	○	○	○	○		34	○	○	○	○
5	○	○	○	○		35	○	○	○	○
6	○	○	○	○		36	○	○	○	○
7	○	○	○	○		37	○	○	○	○
8	○	○	○	○		38	○	○	○	○
9	○	○	○	○		39	○	○	○	○
10	○	○	○	○		40	○	○	○	○
11	○	○	○	○		41	○	○	○	○
12	○	○	○	○		42	○	○	○	○
13	○	○	○	○		43	○	○	○	○
14	○	○	○	○						
15	○	○	○	○						
16	○	○	○	○						
17	○	○	○	○						
18	○	○	○	○						
19	○	○	○	○						
20	○	○	○	○						
21	○	○	○	○						
22	○	○	○	○						
23	○	○	○	○						
24	○	○	○	○						
25	○	○	○	○						
26	○	○	○	○						
27	○	○	○	○						
28	○	○	○	○						
29	○	○	○	○						
30	○	○	○	○						

Key: **D/A** = dimensional analysis
R/P = ratio and proportion

Answers

1 Correct answer — **C**

D/A

$$\frac{1}{300}\ \cancel{gr} \times \frac{1\ ml}{\frac{1}{150}\ \cancel{gr}} = \frac{1\ ml}{300/150} = \frac{1\ ml}{2} = 0.5\ ml$$

R/P

$$\frac{1}{150}\ gr : 1\ ml :: \frac{1}{300}\ gr : x\ ml$$
$$\frac{1}{150}x = \frac{1}{300}$$
$$x = \frac{\frac{1}{300}}{\frac{1}{150}}$$
$$x = 0.5\ ml$$

2 Correct answer — **A**

D/A

$$500\ \cancel{mg} \times \frac{1\ \cancel{g}}{1,000\ \cancel{mg}} \times \frac{6\ ml}{6\ \cancel{g}} = \frac{3,000\ ml}{6,000} = 0.5\ ml$$

R/P

Step 1: Change milligrams to grams.
$$1,000\ mg : 1\ g :: 500\ mg : x\ g$$
$$1,000x = 500$$
$$x = \frac{500}{1,000}$$
$$x = 0.5\ g$$

Step 2: Calculate required milliliters.
$$6\ g : 6\ ml :: 0.5\ g : x\ ml$$
$$6x = 6 \times 0.5$$
$$6x = 3$$
$$x = \frac{3}{6}$$
$$x = 0.5\ ml$$

3 Correct answer — **B**

D/A

$$0.125\ \cancel{mg} \times \frac{1\ ml}{0.25\ \cancel{mg}} = \frac{0.125\ ml}{0.25} = 0.5\ ml$$

R/P

$$0.25\ mg : 1\ ml :: 0.125\ mg : x\ ml$$
$$0.25x = 0.125$$
$$x = \frac{0.125}{0.25}$$
$$x = 0.5\ ml$$

4 Correct answer—**B**

D/A

$$50 \cancel{kg} \times \frac{2 \text{ m\cancel{g}}}{1 \cancel{kg}} \times \frac{10 \text{ ml}}{100 \text{ m\cancel{g}}} = \frac{1{,}000 \text{ ml}}{100} = 10 \text{ ml}$$

R/P

Step 1: Change kilograms to milligrams.
$$1 \text{ kg} : 2 \text{ mg} :: 50 \text{ kg} : x \text{ mg}$$
$$x = 2 \times 50$$
$$x = 100 \text{ mg}$$

Step 2: Calculate required milliliters.

Because 10 ml of the drug equals 100 mg, prepare 10 ml.

5 Correct answer—**D**

D/A

$$60 \cancel{kg} \times \frac{15 \text{ m\cancel{cg}}}{1 \cancel{kg}} \times \frac{1 \text{ m\cancel{g}}}{1{,}000 \text{ m\cancel{cg}}} \times \frac{1 \text{ ml}}{0.5 \text{ m\cancel{g}}} = \frac{900 \text{ ml}}{500} = 1.8 \text{ ml}$$

R/P

Step 1: Change kilograms to micrograms.
$$1 \text{ kg} : 15 \text{ mcg} :: 60 \text{ kg} : x \text{ mcg}$$
$$x = 15 \times 60$$
$$x = 900 \text{ mcg}$$

Step 2: Change micrograms to milligrams.
$$1{,}000 \text{ mcg} : 1 \text{ mg} :: 900 \text{ mcg} : x \text{ mg}$$
$$1000x = 900$$
$$x = \frac{900}{1{,}000}$$
$$x = 0.9 \text{ mg}$$

Step 3: Calculate required milliliters.
$$0.5 \text{ mg} : 1 \text{ ml} :: 0.9 \text{ mg} : x \text{ ml}$$
$$0.5x = 0.9$$
$$x = \frac{0.9}{0.5}$$
$$x = 1.8 \text{ ml}$$

6 Correct answer—**A**

D/A

$$\cancel{100} \cancel{IU} \times \frac{1 \text{ ml}}{\cancel{200} \cancel{IU}} = \frac{1 \text{ ml}}{2} = 0.5 \text{ ml}$$

R/P

$$200 \text{ IU} : 1 \text{ ml} :: 100 \text{ IU} : x \text{ ml}$$
$$200x = 100$$
$$x = \frac{100}{200}$$
$$x = 0.5 \text{ ml}$$

7 Correct answer — **C**

D/A

$$500 \cancel{\text{ mg}} \times \frac{1 \text{ ml}}{400 \cancel{\text{ mg}}} = \frac{5 \text{ ml}}{4} = 1.25 \text{ ml}$$

R/P

$$400 \text{ mg} : 1 \text{ ml} :: 500 \text{ mg} : x \text{ ml}$$
$$400x = 500$$
$$x = \frac{500}{400}$$
$$x = 1.25 \text{ ml}$$

8 Correct answer — **C**

D/A

$$0.25 \cancel{g} \times \frac{1,000 \cancel{\text{ mg}}}{1 \cancel{g}} \times \frac{1 \text{ ml}}{125 \cancel{\text{ mg}}} = \frac{250 \text{ ml}}{125} = 2 \text{ ml}$$

R/P

Step 1: Change grams to milligrams.
$$1 \text{ g} : 1,000 \text{ mg} :: 0.25 \text{ g} : x \text{ mg}$$
$$x = 1,000 \times 0.25$$
$$x = 250 \text{ mg}$$

Step 2: Calculate required milliliters.
$$125 \text{ mg} : 1 \text{ ml} :: 250 \text{ mg} : x \text{ ml}$$
$$125x = 250$$
$$x = \frac{250}{125}$$
$$x = 2 \text{ ml}$$

9 Correct answer — **B**

D/A

$$40 \cancel{\text{ mEq}} \times \frac{1 \text{ ml}}{2 \cancel{\text{ mEq}}} = \frac{40 \text{ ml}}{2} = 20 \text{ ml}$$

R/P

$$2 \text{ mEq} : 1 \text{ ml} :: 40 \text{ mEq} :: x \text{ ml}$$
$$2x = 40$$
$$x = \frac{40}{2}$$
$$x = 20 \text{ ml}$$

10

Correct answer—**D**

D/A

$$1,\cancel{200,000} \, \cancel{U} \times \frac{\cancel{10} \text{ ml}}{6,\cancel{000,000} \, \cancel{U}} = \frac{12 \text{ ml}}{6} = 2 \text{ ml}$$

R/P

$$6,000,000 \text{ U} : 10 \text{ ml} :: 1,200,000 \text{ U} : x \text{ ml}$$
$$6,000,000x = 10 \times 1,200,000$$
$$x = \frac{12,000,000}{6,000,000}$$
$$x = 2 \text{ ml}$$

11

Correct answer—**A**
Remember: 1,000 mg = 1 g

D/A

$$0.02 \, \cancel{g} \times \frac{1,000 \, \cancel{mg}}{1 \, \cancel{g}} \times \frac{1 \text{ ml}}{20 \, \cancel{mg}} = \frac{20 \text{ ml}}{20} = 1 \text{ ml}$$

R/P

Step 1: Change grams to milligrams.
$$1 \text{ g} : 1,000 \text{ mg} :: 0.02 \text{ g} : x \text{ mg}$$
$$x = 1,000 \times 0.02$$
$$x = 20 \text{ mg}$$

Step 2: Calculate required milliliters.

Because vial reads 20 mg = 1 ml, then 0.02 g = 1 ml.

12

Correct answer—**C**

D/A

$$100 \, \cancel{mg} \times \frac{1 \, \cancel{g}}{1,000 \, \cancel{mg}} \times \frac{5 \text{ ml}}{1.1 \, \cancel{g}} = \frac{500 \text{ ml}}{1,100} = 0.45 \text{ ml}$$

R/P

Step 1: Change milligrams to grams.

$$1{,}000 \text{ mg} : 1 \text{ g} :: 100 \text{ mg} : x \text{ g}$$
$$1{,}000x = 100$$
$$x = \frac{100}{1{,}000}$$
$$x = 0.1 \text{ g}$$

Step 2: Calculate required milliliters.

$$1.1 \text{ g} : 5 \text{ ml} :: 0.1 \text{ g} : x \text{ ml}$$
$$1.1x = 5 \times 0.1$$
$$1.1x = 0.5$$
$$x = \frac{0.5}{1.1}$$
$$x = 0.45 \text{ ml}$$

---

13 Correct answer—D

D/A

$$\frac{1}{2} \text{ gr} \times \frac{4 \text{ mg}}{1 \text{ gr}} \times \frac{1 \text{ ml}}{1 \text{ mg}} = \frac{4 \text{ ml}}{2} = 2 \text{ ml}$$

R/P

Step 1: Change grains to milligrams.

$$1 \text{ gr} : 60 \text{ mg} :: \frac{1}{2} \text{ gr} : x \text{ mg}$$
$$x = 60 \times \frac{1}{2}$$
$$x = 30 \text{ mg}$$

Step 2: Calculate required milliliters.

$$15 \text{ mg} : 1 \text{ ml} :: 30 \text{ mg} : x \text{ ml}$$
$$15x = 30$$
$$x = \frac{30}{15}$$
$$x = 2 \text{ ml}$$

---

14 Correct answer—C

D/A

$$7{,}500 \text{ U} \times \frac{1 \text{ ml}}{5{,}000 \text{ U}} = \frac{75 \text{ ml}}{50} = 1.5 \text{ ml}$$

R/P

$$5{,}000 \text{ U} : 1 \text{ ml} :: 7{,}500 \text{ U} : x \text{ ml}$$
$$5{,}000x = 7{,}500$$
$$x = \frac{7{,}500}{5{,}000}$$
$$x = 1.5 \text{ ml}$$

15 Correct answer—**C**

Remember: 30 ℳ = 2 ml

D/A

$$2,500 \, U \times \frac{1 \, ml}{5,000 \, U} \times \frac{30 \, ℳ}{2 \, ml} = \frac{75 \, ℳ}{10} = 7.5 \, ℳ$$

R/P

Step 1: Calculate required milliliters.

$$5,000 \, U : 1 \, ml :: 2,500 \, U : x \, ml$$
$$5,000x = 2,500$$
$$x = \frac{2,500}{5,000}$$
$$x = 0.5 \, ml$$

Step 2: Calculate required minims.

$$2 \, ml : 30 \, ℳ :: 0.5 \, ml : x \, ℳ$$
$$2x = 30 \times 0.5$$
$$2x = 15$$
$$x = \frac{15}{2}$$
$$x = 7.5 \, ℳ$$

16 Correct answer—**D**

D/A

$$0.2 \, g \times \frac{1,000 \, mg}{1 \, g} \times \frac{1 \, ml}{100 \, mg} = \frac{200 \, ml}{100} = 2 \, ml$$

R/P

Step 1: Change grams to millligrams.

$$1 \, g : 1,000 \, mg :: 0.2 \, g : x \, mg$$
$$x = 1,000 \times 0.2$$
$$x = 200 \, mg$$

Step 2: Calculate required milliliters.

$$100 \, mg : 1 \, ml :: 200 \, mg : x \, ml$$
$$100x = 200$$
$$x = \frac{200}{100}$$
$$x = 2 \, ml$$

17 Correct answer—**B**

D/A

$$0.5 \, g \times \frac{10 \, ml}{10 \, g} = \frac{5 \, ml}{10} = 0.5 \, ml$$

R/P

$$10 \text{ g} : 10 \text{ ml} :: 0.5 \text{ g} : x \text{ ml}$$
$$10x = 10 \times 0.5$$
$$x = \frac{5}{10}$$
$$x = 0.5 \text{ ml}$$

18 Correct answer — C

D/A

$$60 \, \cancel{U} \times \frac{1 \text{ ml}}{100 \, \cancel{U}} = \frac{60 \text{ ml}}{100} = 0.6 \text{ ml}$$

R/P

$$100 \text{ U} : 1 \text{ ml} :: 60 \text{ U} : x \text{ ml}$$
$$100x = 60$$
$$x = \frac{60}{100}$$
$$x = 0.6 \text{ ml}$$

19 Correct answer — D

D/A

$$\frac{1}{100} \, \cancel{gr} \times \frac{1 \text{ ml}}{\frac{1}{150} \, \cancel{gr}} = \frac{1 \text{ ml}}{100/150} = \frac{150 \text{ ml}}{100} = 1.5 \text{ ml}$$

R/P

$$\tfrac{1}{150} \text{ gr} : 1 \text{ ml} :: \tfrac{1}{100} \text{ gr} : x \text{ ml}$$
$$\tfrac{1}{150}x = \tfrac{1}{100}$$
$$x = \frac{\frac{1}{100}}{\frac{1}{150}}$$
$$x = \frac{150}{100}$$
$$x = 1.5 \text{ ml}$$

20 Correct answer — C

D/A

$$0.25 \, \cancel{g} \times \frac{2 \text{ ml}}{1 \, \cancel{g}} = 0.5 \text{ ml}$$

R/P

$$1 \text{ g} : 2 \text{ ml} :: 0.25 \text{ g} : x \text{ ml}$$
$$x = 2 \times 0.25$$
$$x = 0.5 \text{ ml}$$

21

Correct answer—**B**

Remember: 15 ♏ = 1 ml

D/A

$$5 \text{ mg} \times \frac{1 \text{ gr}}{60 \text{ mg}} \times \frac{1 \text{ ml}}{\frac{1}{10} \text{ gr}} \times \frac{15 \text{ ♏}}{1 \text{ ml}} = \frac{75 \text{ ♏}}{6} = 12.5 \text{ or } 13 \text{ ♏}$$

R/P

Step 1: Change milligrams to grains.

$$60 \text{ mg}: 1 \text{ gr} :: 5 \text{ mg} : x \text{ gr}$$
$$60x = 5$$
$$x = \frac{5}{60}$$
$$x = \frac{1}{12} \text{ gr}$$

Step 2: Calculate required minims.

$$\frac{1}{10} \text{ gr} : 15 \text{ ♏} :: \frac{1}{12} \text{ gr} : x \text{ ♏}$$
$$\frac{1}{10}x = 15 \times \frac{1}{12}$$
$$x = \frac{15}{12} \times 10$$
$$x = 12.5 \text{ or } 13 \text{ ♏}$$

22

Correct answer—**B**

D/A

$$0.1 \text{ g} \times \frac{1{,}000 \text{ mg}}{1 \text{ g}} \times \frac{1 \text{ ml}}{50 \text{ mg}} = \frac{100 \text{ ml}}{50} = 2 \text{ ml}$$

R/P

Step 1: Change grams to milligrams.

$$1 \text{ g} : 1{,}000 \text{ mg} :: 0.1 \text{ g} : x \text{ mg}$$
$$x = 1{,}000 \times 0.1$$
$$x = 100 \text{ mg}$$

Step 2: Calculate required milliliters.

$$50 \text{ mg} : 1 \text{ ml} :: 100 \text{ mg} : x \text{ ml}$$
$$50x = 100$$
$$x = \frac{100}{50}$$
$$x = 2 \text{ ml}$$

23

Correct answer—**B**

D/A

$$0.1 \text{ g} \times \frac{1{,}000 \text{ mg}}{1 \text{ g}} \times \frac{1 \text{ ml}}{100 \text{ mg}} = \frac{100 \text{ ml}}{100} = 1 \text{ ml}$$

R/P

Step 1: Change grams to milligrams.
$$1 \text{ g} : 1{,}000 \text{ mg} :: 0.1 \text{ g} : x \text{ mg}$$
$$x = 1{,}000 \times 0.1$$
$$x = 100 \text{ mg}$$

Step 2: Calculate required milliliters.

Because drug is available as 100 mg/ml, give 1 ml.

24 Correct answer — **C**

D/A

$$1.5 \text{ m}^2 \times \frac{6 \text{ mg}}{1 \text{ m}^2} \times \frac{1 \text{ ml}}{10 \text{ mg}} = \frac{9 \text{ ml}}{10} = 0.9 \text{ ml}$$

R/P

Step 1: Calculate required milligrams.
$$1 \text{ m}^2 : 6 \text{ mg} :: 1.5 \text{ m}^2 : x \text{ mg}$$
$$x = 6 \times 1.5$$
$$x = 9 \text{ mg}$$

Step 2: Calculate required milliliters.
$$10 \text{ mg} : 1 \text{ ml} :: 9 \text{ mg} : x \text{ ml}$$
$$10x = 9$$
$$x = \frac{9}{10}$$
$$x = 0.9 \text{ ml}$$

25 Correct answer — **A**

Remember: 1 g = 1,000 mg; 1:10,000 = 1 g in 10,000 ml

D/A

$$0.5 \text{ mg} \times \frac{10{,}000 \text{ ml}}{1{,}000 \text{ mg}} = 5 \text{ ml}$$

R/P

$$1{,}000 \text{ mg} : 10{,}000 \text{ ml} :: 0.5 \text{ mg} : x \text{ ml}$$
$$1{,}000x = 10{,}000 \times 0.5$$
$$x = \frac{5{,}000}{1{,}000}$$
$$x = 5 \text{ ml}$$

26 Correct answer — **C**

D/A

$$1.2 \text{ mg} \times \frac{1 \text{ ml}}{0.4 \text{ mg}} = \frac{1.2 \text{ ml}}{0.4} = 3 \text{ ml}$$

R/P

$$0.4 \text{ mg} : 1 \text{ ml} :: 1.2 \text{ mg} : x \text{ ml}$$
$$0.4x = 1.2$$
$$x = \frac{1.2}{0.4}$$
$$x = 3 \text{ ml}$$

27 Correct answer—**B**

D/A

$$\frac{1}{200} \cancel{gr} \times \frac{60 \cancel{mg}}{1 \cancel{gr}} \times \frac{1 \text{ ml}}{0.3 \cancel{mg}} = \frac{60 \text{ ml}}{60} = 1 \text{ ml}$$

R/P

Step 1: Change grains to milligrams.
$$1 \text{ gr} : 60 \text{ mg} :: \frac{1}{200} \text{ gr} : x \text{ mg}$$
$$x = 60 \times \frac{1}{200}$$
$$x = 0.3 \text{ mg}$$

Step 2: Calculate required milliliters.

Because 1 ml = 0.3 mg, give 1 ml.

28 Correct answer—**C**

D/A

$$5 \cancel{U} \times \frac{1 \text{ ml}}{10 \cancel{U}} = \frac{5 \text{ ml}}{10} = 0.5 \text{ ml}$$

R/P

$$10 \text{ U} : 1 \text{ ml} :: 5 \text{ U} : x \text{ ml}$$
$$10x = 5$$
$$x = \frac{5}{10}$$
$$x = 0.5 \text{ ml}$$

29 Correct answer—**D**

D/A

$$1.3 \cancel{m^2} \times \frac{1.4 \cancel{mg}}{1 \cancel{m^2}} \times \frac{0.5 \text{ ml}}{1 \cancel{mg}} = 0.91 \text{ or } 0.9 \text{ ml}$$

R/P

Step 1: Calculate required milligrams.
$$1 \text{ m}^2 : 1.4 \text{ mg} :: 1.3 \text{ m}^2 : x \text{ mg}$$
$$x = 1.4 \times 1.3$$
$$x = 1.82 \text{ mg}$$

Step 2: Calculate required milliliters.
$$1 \text{ mg} : 0.5 \text{ ml} :: 1.82 \text{ mg} : x \text{ ml}$$
$$x = 0.5 \times 1.82$$
$$x = 0.91 \text{ or } 0.9 \text{ ml}$$

30

Correct answer — **B**

Remember: 1 ml = 15 ℥

D/A

$$1.7 \text{ m}^2 \times \frac{100 \text{ U}}{1 \text{ m}^2} \times \frac{1 \text{ ml}}{200 \text{ U}} \times \frac{15 \text{ ℥}}{1 \text{ ml}} = \frac{25.5 \text{ ℥}}{200} = 12.75 \text{ or } 13 \text{ ℥}$$

R/P

Step 1: Calculate required units.
$$1 \text{ m}^2 : 100 \text{ U} :: 1.7 \text{ m}^2 : x \text{ U}$$
$$x = 100 \times 1.7$$
$$x = 170 \text{ U}$$

Step 2: Calculate required minims.
$$200 \text{ U} : 15 \text{ ℥} :: 170 \text{ U} : x \text{ ℥}$$
$$200x = 170 \times 15$$
$$x = \frac{2,550}{200}$$
$$x = 12.75 \text{ or } 13 \text{ ℥}$$

31

Correct answer — **D**

D/A

$$60 \text{ kg} \times \frac{0.5 \text{ mg}}{1 \text{ kg}} \times \frac{1 \text{ ℥}}{1 \text{ mg}} \times \frac{1 \text{ ml}}{15 \text{ ℥}} = \frac{30 \text{ ml}}{15} = 2 \text{ ml}$$

R/P

Step 1: Change kilograms to milligrams.
$$1 \text{ kg} : 0.5 \text{ mg} :: 60 \text{ kg} : x \text{ mg}$$
$$x = 0.5 \times 60$$
$$x = 30 \text{ mg}$$

Step 2: Calculate required minims.

Because 1 mg = 1 ℥, then 30 mg = 30 ℥.

Step 3: Change minims to milliliters.
$$15 \text{ ℥} : 1 \text{ ml} :: 30 \text{ ℥} : x \text{ ml}$$
$$15x = 30$$
$$x = \frac{30}{15}$$
$$x = 2 \text{ ml}$$

32 Correct answer—**D**

D/A

$$45 \text{ kg} \times \frac{10 \text{ mg}}{1 \text{ kg}} \times \frac{1 \text{ ml}}{130 \text{ mg}} = \frac{450 \text{ ml}}{130} = 3.46 \text{ or } 3.5 \text{ ml}$$

R/P

Step 1: Change kilograms to milligrams.

$$1 \text{ kg} : 10 \text{ mg} :: 45 \text{ kg} : x \text{ mg}$$
$$x = 10 \times 45$$
$$x = 450 \text{ mg}$$

Step 2: Calculate required milliliters.

$$130 \text{ mg} : 1 \text{ ml} :: 450 \text{ mg} : x \text{ ml}$$
$$130x = 450$$
$$x = \frac{450}{130}$$
$$x = 3.46 \text{ or } 3.5 \text{ ml}$$

33 Correct answer—**C**

Remember: 1 ml = 15 ♏

D/A

$$50 \text{ kg} \times \frac{0.07 \text{ mg}}{1 \text{ kg}} \times \frac{1 \text{ ml}}{5 \text{ mg}} \times \frac{15 \text{ ♏}}{1 \text{ ml}} = \frac{52.5 \text{ ♏}}{5} = 10.5 \text{ or } 11 \text{ ♏}$$

R/P

Step 1: Change kilograms to milligrams.

$$1 \text{ kg} : 0.07 \text{ mg} :: 50 \text{ kg} : x \text{ mg}$$
$$x = 0.07 \times 50$$
$$x = 3.5 \text{ mg}$$

Step 2: Calculate required minims.

$$5 \text{ mg} : 15 \text{ ♏} :: 3.5 \text{ mg} : x \text{ ♏}$$
$$5x = 15 \times 3.5$$
$$x = \frac{52.5}{5}$$
$$x = 10.5 \text{ or } 11 \text{ ♏}$$

34 Correct answer—**B**

D/A

$$50 \text{ mg} \times \frac{2 \text{ ml}}{125 \text{ mg}} = \frac{100 \text{ ml}}{125} = 0.8 \text{ ml}$$

R/P

$$125 \text{ mg} : 2 \text{ ml} :: 50 \text{ mg} : x \text{ ml}$$
$$125x = 2 \times 50$$
$$x = \frac{100}{125}$$
$$x = 0.8 \text{ ml}$$

35 Correct answer — **A**

D/A

$$0.4 \cancel{g} \times \frac{1{,}000 \cancel{mg}}{1 \cancel{g}} \times \frac{1 \text{ ml}}{250 \cancel{mg}} = \frac{400 \text{ ml}}{250} = 1.6 \text{ ml}$$

R/P

Step 1: Change grams to milligrams.
$$1 \text{ g} : 1{,}000 \text{ mg} :: 0.4 \text{ g} : x \text{ mg}$$
$$x = 1{,}000 \times 0.4$$
$$x = 400 \text{ mg}$$

Step 2: Calculate required milliliters.
$$250 \text{ mg} : 1 \text{ ml} :: 400 \text{ mg} : x \text{ ml}$$
$$250x = 400$$
$$x = \frac{400}{250}$$
$$x = 1.6 \text{ ml}$$

36 Correct answer — **C**

D/A

$$500 \cancel{mg} \times \frac{1 \text{ ml}}{330 \cancel{mg}} = \frac{500 \text{ ml}}{330} = 1.51 \text{ or } 1.5 \text{ ml}$$

R/P

$$330 \text{ mg} : 1 \text{ ml} :: 500 \text{ mg} : x \text{ ml}$$
$$330x = 500$$
$$x = \frac{500}{330}$$
$$x = 1.51 \text{ or } 1.5 \text{ ml}$$

37 Correct answer — **D**

D/A

$$55 \cancel{kg} \times \frac{10{,}000 \cancel{U}}{1 \cancel{kg}} \times \frac{1 \text{ ml}}{50{,}000 \cancel{U}} = \frac{55 \text{ ml}}{5} = 11 \text{ ml}$$

R/P

Step 1: Calculate required units.
$$1 \text{ kg} : 10{,}000 \text{ U} :: 55 \text{ kg} : x \text{ U}$$
$$x = 10{,}000 \times 55$$
$$x = 550{,}000 \text{ U}$$

Step 2: Calculate required milliliters.

$$50,000 \text{ U} : 1 \text{ ml} :: 550,000 \text{ U} : x \text{ ml}$$
$$50,000x = 550,000$$
$$x = \frac{550,000}{50,000}$$
$$x = 11 \text{ ml}$$

38 Correct answer—**A**

Remember: 0.5% solution is 0.5 g in 100 ml.

D/A

$$250 \text{ ml} \times \frac{0.5 \text{ g}}{100 \text{ ml}} = \frac{125 \text{ g}}{100} = 1.25 \text{ g}$$

R/P

$$100 \text{ ml} : 0.5 \text{ g} :: 250 \text{ ml} : x \text{ g}$$
$$100x = 0.5 \text{ g} \times 250$$
$$x = \frac{125}{100}$$
$$x = 1.25 \text{ g}$$

39 Correct answer—**A**

D/A

$$\frac{5 \text{ g}}{250 \text{ ml}} = \frac{1}{50} \text{ or } \frac{2}{100} = 2\%$$

R/P

$$250 \text{ ml} : 5 \text{ g} :: 100 \text{ ml} : x \text{ g}$$
$$250x = 5 \times 100$$
$$x = \frac{500}{250}$$
$$x = 2 \text{ g}$$
$$2 \text{ g}/100 \text{ ml} = 2\%$$

40 Correct answer—**D**

D/A

$$2,000 \text{ ml} \times \frac{0.9 \text{ g}}{100 \text{ ml}} = 18 \text{ g}$$

R/P

$$100 \text{ ml} : 0.9 \text{ g} :: 2,000 \text{ ml} : x \text{ g}$$
$$100x = 0.9 \times 2,000$$
$$x = \frac{1,800}{100}$$
$$x = 18 \text{ g}$$

41

Correct answer — **A**

Remember: 500 mg = 0.5 g

D/A

$$0.5\ \cancel{g} \times \frac{100\ \text{ml}}{\cancel{50}\ \cancel{g}} = \frac{5\ \text{ml}}{5} = 1\ \text{ml}$$

R/P

$$50\ g : 100\ ml :: 0.5\ g : x\ ml$$
$$50x = 100 \times 0.5$$
$$x = \frac{50}{50}$$
$$x = 1\ ml$$

42

Correct answer — **C**

D/A

$$50\ \cancel{ml} \times \frac{\overset{1}{\cancel{25}}\ g}{\underset{4}{\cancel{100}}\ \cancel{ml}} = \frac{50\ g}{4} = 12.5\ g$$

R/P

$$100\ ml : 25\ g :: 50\ ml : x\ g$$
$$100x = 25 \times 50$$
$$x = \frac{1,250}{100}$$
$$x = 12.5\ g$$

43

Correct answer — **C**

D/A

$$120\ \cancel{ml} \times \frac{25\ ml}{\cancel{100}\ \cancel{ml}} = \frac{300}{10} = 30\ ml$$

R/P

$$100\ ml : 25\ ml :: 120\ ml : x\ ml$$
$$100x = 25 \times 120$$
$$100x = 3,000$$
$$x = \frac{3,000}{100}$$
$$x = 30\ ml$$

CHAPTER 6

Pediatric Dosages

Questions

1 A 9-kg infant is to receive penicillin V (V-Cillin) 15 mg/kg P.O. How many milligrams of this antibiotic should the nurse administer?

A. 115 mg
B. 135 mg
C. 182 mg
D. 250 mg

2 How many milligrams of medication should be administered to a child weighing 40 lb if the order calls for 20 mg/kg?

A. 100 mg
B. 250 mg
C. 364 mg
D. 480 mg

3 The physician prescribes the antipyretic acetaminophen (Tylenol) for a child who weighs 15 kg. What would be the correct dose if the order were 3 mg/kg P.O.?

A. 45 mg
B. 50 mg
C. 52 mg
D. 68 mg

4 What is the correct dose of digoxin (Lanoxin), a cardiac glycoside, for a 3-month-old infant weighing 5.4 kg when the order reads 0.035 mg/kg P.O.?

A. 0.19 mg
B. 0.25 mg
C. 25 mg
D. 57 mg

5 A 4-year-old child weighing 30 lb is to receive atropine sulfate, an anticholinergic drug. Which dose should the nurse administer if the order reads 0.01 mg/kg S.C.?

A. 0.06 mg
B. 0.08 mg
C. 0.12 mg
D. 0.14 mg

6 The antihistamine diphenhydramine (Benadryl) has been prescribed for a child weighing 36 lb. The bottle label reads: 1 ml = 5 mg. How many milliliters should the nurse prepare if the order reads 1.25 mg/kg P.O.?

A. 0.19 ml
B. 1.6 ml
C. 3 ml
D. 4.1 ml

7 A 10-year-old child weighing 30 kg requires intramuscular vitamin B_{12} (Cyanocobalamin) therapy. What is the dose if the order reads 2 mcg/kg?

A. 20 mcg
B. 60 mcg
C. 90 mcg
D. 125 mcg

8 Phenobarbital (Luminal), an anticonvulsant, has been prescribed for a child weighing 44 lb. The recommended oral dose is 5 mg/kg. How many milligrams should the nurse administer?

A. 10 mg
B. 25 mg
C. 76 mg
D. 100 mg

9 A child weighing 15 kg must receive the antibiotic tobramycin sulfate (Nebcin) I.M. What is the dose for this child if the recommended amount is 3 mg/kg?

A. 0.2 mg
B. 1.25 mg
C. 45 mg
D. 92 mg

10 The oral sulfonamide sulfisoxazole (Gantrisin) has been ordered for a child weighing 20 kg. How many milligrams should the nurse administer if the order reads 30 mg/kg?

A. 148 mg
B. 250 mg
C. 485 mg
D. 600 mg

11 A child weighing 50 lb must receive methylphenidate (Ritalin) therapy. What would be the safe dose of this central nervous system stimulant if the recommended optimum daily dose is 2 mg/kg P.O.?

A. 22 mg
B. 45 mg
C. 90 mg
D. 224 mg

12 A child weighing 38 kg is being treated for active tuberculosis with oral rifampin (Rifadin). The recommended dose for this antitubercular drug is 10 mg/kg. Which dose is considered safe for this child?

A. 275 mg
B. 300 mg
C. 380 mg
D. 410.5 mg

13 Phenazopyridine (Pyridium), a urinary antiseptic, is ordered for a child who weighs 42 lb. Which dose should the nurse should administer if the recommended dose is 4 mg/kg P.O.?

A. 76 mg
B. 83.8 mg
C. 139 mg
D. 174.5 mg

14 The antineoplastic vincristine (Oncovin) is ordered for a child with a body surface area (BSA) of 0.6 m^2. The recommended dose is 1.5 mg/m^2 I.V. weekly. How many milligrams should the nurse administer?

A. 0.45 mg
B. 0.61 mg
C. 0.9 mg
D. 1.44 mg

15 The physician orders acyclovir sodium (Zovirax), 250 mg/m^2 I.V. infusion over 1 hour. How many milligrams of this antiviral drug should the nurse administer to a child whose BSA is 0.5 m^2?

A. 25 mg
B. 100 mg
C. 115 mg
D. 125 mg

16 An I.V. bolus of atropine sulfate, 0.3 mg/m², has been ordered for a child with a BSA of 0.46 m². How many milligrams of this anticholinergic should the nurse administer?

A. 0.04 mg
B. 0.14 mg
C. 2 mg
D. 3 mg

17 The physician orders 3.3 mg/m² of the oral form of methotrexate (Folex), an antineoplastic, for a patient whose BSA is 0.9 m². Which dose is correct?

A. 3 mg
B. 3.7 mg
C. 10.2 mg
D. 12.5 mg

18 A 5-year-old child is being treated for diarrhea. How many milliliters of the oral kaolin and pectin mixture (Kaopectate) are safe for this child when the adult dose is 4 Tbs?

A. 1.5 ml
B. 3.6 ml
C. 12 ml
D. 24 ml

19 The nurse is ordered to administer the laxative magnesium hydroxide (Milk of Magnesia) P.O. to a 7-year-old child. The recommended adult dose is 30 ml. How many milliliters should the nurse administer?

A. 12 ml
B. 17 ml
C. 20 ml
D. 32 ml

20 An I.V. bolus of the antiarrhythmic isoproterenol (Isuprel) is ordered for a 3½-year-old child. The adult dose is 0.03 mg. Which dose is safe for this child?

A. 0.004 mg
B. 0.008 mg
C. 1 mg
D. 1.33 mg

21 The physician prescribes a dose of the emetic ipecac syrup for a 10-month-old infant. The adult dose is 15 ml P.O. How many minims should the nurse administer?

A. 1 ℔
B. 14 ℔
C. 15 ℔
D. 20 ℔

Answer sheet

	A	B	C	D
1	○	○	○	○
2	○	○	○	○
3	○	○	○	○
4	○	○	○	○
5	○	○	○	○
6	○	○	○	○
7	○	○	○	○
8	○	○	○	○
9	○	○	○	○
10	○	○	○	○
11	○	○	○	○
12	○	○	○	○
13	○	○	○	○
14	○	○	○	○
15	○	○	○	○
16	○	○	○	○
17	○	○	○	○
18	○	○	○	○
19	○	○	○	○
20	○	○	○	○
21	○	○	○	○

Answers

1 Correct answer — **B**

D/A

$$9 \text{ kg} \times \frac{15 \text{ mg}}{1 \text{ kg}} = 135 \text{ mg}$$

R/P

$$1 \text{ kg} : 15 \text{ mg} :: 9 \text{ kg} : x \text{ mg}$$
$$x = 15 \times 9$$
$$x = 135 \text{ mg}$$

2 Correct answer — **C**

D/A

$$40 \text{ lb} \times \frac{1 \text{ kg}}{2.2 \text{ lb}} \times \frac{20 \text{ mg}}{1 \text{ kg}} = \frac{800 \text{ mg}}{2.2} = 363.6 \text{ or } 364 \text{ mg}$$

R/P

Step 1: Change pounds to kilograms.
$$2.2 \text{ lb} : 1 \text{ kg} :: 40 \text{ lb} : x \text{ kg}$$
$$2.2x = 40$$
$$x = \frac{40}{2.2}$$
$$x = 18.18 \text{ kg}$$

Step 2: Calculate required milligrams.
$$1 \text{ kg} : 20 \text{ mg} :: 18.18 \text{ kg} : x \text{ mg}$$
$$x = 20 \times 18.18$$
$$x = 363.6 \text{ or } 364 \text{ mg}$$

3 Correct answer — **A**

D/A

$$15 \text{ kg} \times \frac{3 \text{ mg}}{1 \text{ kg}} = 45 \text{ mg}$$

R/P

$$1 \text{ kg} : 3 \text{ mg} :: 15 \text{ kg} : x \text{ mg}$$
$$x = 3 \times 15$$
$$x = 45 \text{ mg}$$

4 Correct answer — **A**

D/A

$$5.4 \text{ kg} \times \frac{0.035 \text{ mg}}{1 \text{ kg}} = 0.189 \text{ or } 0.19 \text{ mg}$$

R/P
$$1 \text{ kg} : 0.035 \text{ mg} :: 5.4 \text{ kg} : x \text{ mg}$$
$$x = 0.035 \times 5.4$$
$$x = 0.189 \text{ or } 0.19 \text{ mg}$$

5 Correct answer — **D**

D/A
$$30 \text{ lb} \times \frac{1 \text{ kg}}{2.2 \text{ lb}} \times \frac{0.01 \text{ mg}}{1 \text{ kg}} = \frac{0.3 \text{ mg}}{2.2} = 0.136 \text{ or } 0.14 \text{ mg}$$

R/P

Step 1 : Change pounds to kilograms.
$$2.2 \text{ lb} : 1 \text{ kg} :: 30 \text{ lb} : x \text{ kg}$$
$$2.2x = 30$$
$$x = \frac{30}{2.2}$$
$$x = 13.6 \text{ kg}$$

Step 2: Calculate required milligrams.
$$1 \text{ kg} : 0.01 \text{ mg} :: 13.6 \text{ kg} : x \text{ mg}$$
$$x = 0.01 \times 13.6$$
$$x = 0.136 \text{ or } 0.14 \text{ mg}$$

6 Correct answer — **D**

D/A
$$36 \text{ lb} \times \frac{1 \text{ kg}}{2.2 \text{ lb}} \times \frac{1.25 \text{ mg}}{1 \text{ kg}} \times \frac{1 \text{ ml}}{5 \text{ mg}} = \frac{45 \text{ ml}}{11} = 4.09 \text{ or } 4.1 \text{ ml}$$

R/P

Step 1: Change pounds to kilograms.
$$2.2 \text{ lb} : 1 \text{ kg} :: 36 \text{ lb} : x \text{ kg}$$
$$2.2x = 36$$
$$x = \frac{36}{2.2}$$
$$x = 16.36 \text{ kg}$$

Step 2: Determine required milligrams.
$$1 \text{ kg} : 1.25 \text{ mg} :: 16.36 \text{ kg} : x \text{ mg}$$
$$x = 1.25 \times 16.36$$
$$x = 20.45 \text{ mg}$$

Step 3: Determine required milliliters.

$$5 \text{ mg} : 1 \text{ ml} :: 20.45 \text{ mg} : x \text{ ml}$$
$$5x = 20.45$$
$$x = \frac{20.45}{5}$$
$$x = 4.09 \text{ or } 4.1 \text{ ml}$$

7 Correct answer — **B**

D/A

$$30 \cancel{\text{ kg}} \times \frac{2 \text{ mcg}}{1 \cancel{\text{ kg}}} = 60 \text{ mcg}$$

R/P

$$1 \text{ kg} : 2 \text{ mcg} :: 30 \text{ kg} : x \text{ mcg}$$
$$x = 2 \times 30$$
$$x = 60 \text{ mcg}$$

8 Correct answer — **D**

D/A

$$44 \cancel{\text{ lb}} \times \frac{1 \cancel{\text{ kg}}}{2.2 \cancel{\text{ lb}}} \times \frac{5 \text{ mg}}{1 \cancel{\text{ kg}}} = \frac{220 \text{ mg}}{2.2} = 100 \text{ mg}$$

R/P

Step 1: Change pounds to kilograms.

$$2.2 \text{ lb} : 1 \text{ kg} :: 44 \text{ lb} : x \text{ kg}$$
$$2.2x = 44$$
$$x = \frac{44}{2.2}$$
$$x = 20 \text{ kg}$$

Step 2: Calculate required milligrams.

$$1 \text{ kg} : 5 \text{ mg} :: 20 \text{ kg} : x \text{ mg}$$
$$x = 5 \times 20$$
$$x = 100 \text{ mg}$$

9 Correct answer — **C**

D/A

$$15 \cancel{\text{ kg}} \times \frac{3 \text{ mg}}{1 \cancel{\text{ kg}}} = 45 \text{ mg}$$

R/P

$$1 \text{ kg} : 3 \text{ mg} :: 15 \text{ kg} : x \text{ mg}$$
$$x = 15 \times 3$$
$$x = 45 \text{ mg}$$

10 Correct answer—**D**

D/A

$$20 \text{ kg} \times \frac{30 \text{ mg}}{1 \text{ kg}} = 600 \text{ mg}$$

R/P

$$1 \text{ kg} : 30 \text{ mg} :: 20 \text{ kg} : x \text{ mg}$$
$$x = 30 \times 20$$
$$x = 600 \text{ mg}$$

11 Correct answer—**B**

D/A

$$50 \text{ lb} \times \frac{1 \text{ kg}}{2.2 \text{ lb}} \times \frac{2 \text{ mg}}{1 \text{ kg}} = \frac{100 \text{ mg}}{2.2} = 45.4 \text{ or } 45 \text{ mg}$$

R/P

Step 1: Change pounds to kilograms.
$$2.2 \text{ lb} : 1 \text{ kg} :: 50 \text{ lb} : x \text{ kg}$$
$$2.2x = 50$$
$$x = \frac{50}{2.2}$$
$$x = 22.72 \text{ kg}$$

Step 2: Calculate required milligrams.
$$1 \text{ kg} : 2 \text{ mg} :: 22.72 \text{ kg} : x \text{ mg}$$
$$x = 2 \times 22.72$$
$$x = 45.4 \text{ or } 45 \text{ mg}$$

12 Correct answer—**C**

D/A

$$38 \text{ kg} \times \frac{10 \text{ mg}}{1 \text{ kg}} = 380 \text{ mg}$$

R/P

$$1 \text{ kg} : 10 \text{ mg} :: 38 \text{ kg} : x \text{ mg}$$
$$x = 10 \times 38$$
$$x = 380 \text{ mg}$$

13 Correct answer — **A**

D/A

$$42 \text{ lb} \times \frac{1 \text{ kg}}{2.2 \text{ lb}} \times \frac{4 \text{ mg}}{1 \text{ kg}} = \frac{168 \text{ mg}}{2.2} = 76.36 \text{ or } 76 \text{ mg}$$

R/P

Step 1: Change pounds to kilograms.

2.2 lb : 1 kg :: 42 lb : x kg

$2.2x = 42$

$$x = \frac{42}{2.2}$$

$x = 19.09$ kg

Step 2: Calculate required milligrams.

1 kg : 4 mg :: 19.09 kg : x mg

$x = 4 \times 19.09$

$x = 76.4$ or 76 mg

14 Correct answer — **C**

D/A

$$0.6 \text{ m}^2 \times \frac{1.5 \text{ mg}}{1 \text{ m}^2} = 0.9 \text{ mg}$$

R/P

1 m² : 1.5 mg :: 0.6 m² : x mg

$x = 1.5 \times 0.6$

$x = 0.9$ mg

15 Correct answer — **D**

D/A

$$0.5 \text{ m}^2 \times \frac{250 \text{ mg}}{1 \text{ m}^2} = 125 \text{ mg}$$

R/P

1 m² : 250 mg :: 0.5 m² : x mg

$x = 250 \times 0.5$

$x = 125$ mg

16 Correct answer — **B**

D/A

$$0.46 \text{ m}^2 \times \frac{0.3 \text{ mg}}{1 \text{ m}^2} = 0.138 \text{ or } 0.14 \text{ mg}$$

R/P

$$1 \text{ m}^2 : 0.3 \text{ mg} :: 0.46 \text{ m}^2 : x \text{ mg}$$
$$x = 0.3 \times 0.46$$
$$x = 0.138 \text{ or } 0.14 \text{ mg}$$

---

17 Correct answer—**A**

D/A

$$0.9 \ \cancel{\text{m}^2} \times \frac{3.3 \text{ mg}}{1 \ \cancel{\text{m}^2}} = 2.97 \text{ or } 3 \text{ mg}$$

R/P

$$1 \text{ m}^2 : 3.3 \text{ mg} :: 0.9 \text{ m}^2 : x \text{ mg}$$
$$x = 3.3 \times 0.9$$
$$x = 2.97 \text{ or } 3 \text{ mg}$$

---

18 Correct answer—**D**

Remember: When figuring dosage based on age, use 150 months as the adult value

D/A

$$\overset{6}{\cancel{60}} \text{ months} \times \frac{4 \ \cancel{\text{Tbs}}}{\underset{10}{\cancel{150}} \text{ months}} \times \frac{\overset{1}{\cancel{15}} \text{ ml}}{1 \ \cancel{\text{Tbs}}} = 24 \text{ ml}$$

R/P

Step 1: Determine required tablespoons.

$$150 \text{ months} : 4 \text{ Tbs} :: 60 \text{ months} : x \text{ Tbs}$$
$$150x = 4 \times 60$$
$$150x = 240$$
$$x = \frac{240}{150}$$
$$x = 1\tfrac{3}{5} \text{ Tbs}$$

Step 2: Change tablespoons to milliliters.

$$1 \text{ Tbs} : 15 \text{ ml} :: 1\tfrac{3}{5} \text{ Tbs} : x \text{ ml}$$
$$x = 15 \times 1\tfrac{3}{5}$$
$$x = 24 \text{ ml}$$

---

19 Correct answer—**B**

D/A

$$84 \ \cancel{\text{months}} \times \frac{\overset{1}{\cancel{30}} \text{ ml}}{\underset{5}{\cancel{150}} \ \cancel{\text{months}}} = \frac{84 \text{ ml}}{5} = 16.8 \text{ or } 17 \text{ ml}$$

R/P

$$150 \text{ months} : 30 \text{ ml} :: 84 \text{ months} : x \text{ ml}$$
$$150x = 30 \times 84$$
$$x = \frac{2{,}520}{150}$$
$$x = 16.8 \text{ or } 17 \text{ ml}$$

20 Correct answer—**B**

D/A

$$42 \text{ months} \times \frac{0.03 \text{ mg}}{150 \text{ months}} = \frac{1.26 \text{ mg}}{150} = 0.008 \text{ mg}$$

R/P

$$150 \text{ months} : 0.03 \text{ mg} :: 42 \text{ months} : x \text{ mg}$$
$$150x = 0.03 \times 42$$
$$x = \frac{1.26}{150}$$
$$x = 0.008 \text{ mg}$$

21 Correct answer—**C**
Remember: 1 ml = 15 ♏

D/A

$$\overset{1}{\cancel{10} \text{ months}} \times \frac{\overset{1}{\cancel{15} \text{ ml}}}{\underset{\cancel{10}}{\cancel{150} \text{ months}}} \times \frac{15 \text{ ♏}}{1 \text{ ml}} = 15 \text{ ♏}$$

R/P

$$150 \text{ months} : 15 \text{ ml} :: 10 \text{ months} : x \text{ ml}$$
$$150x = 15 \times 10$$
$$x = \frac{150}{150}$$
$$x = 1 \text{ ml or } 15 \text{ ♏}$$

CHAPTER 7

Intravenous Therapy

Questions

1 The physician's order reads "Infuse 1,500 ml of D₅W in 12 hours."
What is the correct flow rate of this isotonic solution when the drop
factor is 15 gtt = 1 ml?

A. 15 gtt/minute
B. 31 gtt/minute
C. 64 gtt/minute
D. 76 gtt/minute

2 A patient is to receive a microdrip infusion of 1,000 ml of normal (0.9%)
saline solution over 24 hours. The drop factor is 60 mcgtt = 1 ml. What is
the correct flow rate?

A. 42 mcgtt/minute
B. 48 mcgtt/minute
C. 72 mcgtt/minute
D. 95 mcgtt/minute

3 At 3 p.m., a patient must receive 1 g of cefazolin (Ancef) intravenous
piggyback (I.V.P.B.) in 150 ml of of dextrose 5% in water (D₅W), to be
infused over 30 minutes. The drop factor is 10 gtt = 1 ml. What is
the correct flow rate for this antibiotic solution?

A. 12 gtt/minute
B. 28 gtt/minute
C. 50 gtt/minute
D. 100 gtt/minute

4 At 9 a.m., a patient has 500 ml of a D₅W solution remaining in an
infusion bag. The infusion must end at 1 p.m., and the drop factor is
20 gtt = 1 ml. What is the correct flow rate?

A. 9 gtt/minute
B. 15 gtt/minute
C. 34 gtt/minute
D. 42 gtt/minute

5 A patient is to receive 125 ml of 5% dextrose in lactated Ringer's
solution in 1½ hours. The drop factor is 60 mcgtt = 1 ml. How many
microdrops per minute should the patient receive?

A. 22 mcgtt/minute
B. 79 mcgtt/minute
C. 83 mcgtt/minute
D. 114 mcgtt/minute

6 The physician orders 2,500 ml of D₅W to infuse over 24 hours. What would be the flow rate of this isotonic solution if the drop factor is 10 gtt = 1 ml?

A. 17 gtt/minute
B. 75 gtt/minute
C. 92 gtt/minute
D. 248 gtt/minute

7 As part of his postoperative regimen, a patient is to receive all of the following hypertonic solutions intravenously within 24 hours: 1,000 ml dextrose 5% in ½ normal saline solution, 1,000 ml dextrose 5% in normal saline solution, and 1,000 ml dextrose 5% in lactated Ringer's solution. If the I.V. tubing has a drop factor of 10 gtt = 1 ml, what is the correct flow rate for this I.V. therapy?

A. 18 gtt/minute
B. 21 gtt/minute
C. 44 gtt/minute
D. 96 gtt/minute

8 The physician orders an infusion of 750 ml of dextrose 5% in ½ normal saline solution over 8 hours. What is the appropriate flow rate for this hypertonic solution when the tubing has a drop factor of 15 gtt = 1 ml?

A. 23 gtt/minute
B. 42 gtt/minute
C. 67 gtt/minute
D. 230 gtt/minute

9 The physician orders 400 ml of hypotonic 2.5% dextrose in water, to be infused in 4 hours. The drop factor is 60 mcgtt = 1 ml. Which flow rate is correct?

A. 60 mcgtt/minute
B. 100 mcgtt/minute
C. 131 mcgtt/minute
D. 189 mcgtt/minute

10 To stabilize a patient's intravascular volume, the physician orders 1,000 ml of hypertonic dextrose 5% in normal saline solution. Available tubing is listed as 10 gtt = 1 ml. What is the correct flow rate if the infusion is for 6 hours?

A. 8 gtt/minute
B. 10 gtt/minute
C. 20 gtt/minute
D. 28 gtt/minute

11 If 500 ml of normal saline solution must be infused in 2 hours and the I.V. tubing has a drop factor of 10 gtt = 1 ml, what is the flow rate for this intravascular volume expander?

A. 1 gtt/minute
B. 15 gtt/minute
C. 27 gtt/minute
D. 42 gtt/minute

12 The physician orders 1 g of cefoxitin sodium (Mefoxin) in 100 ml of D_5W, to be infused over 60 minutes. What is the correct flow rate for this cephalosporin antibiotic when the tubing drop factor is listed as 60 mcgtt = 1 ml?

A. 100 mcgtt/minute
B. 110 mcgtt/minute
C. 125 mcgtt/minute
D. 135 mcgtt/minute

13 The physician's order reads "Infuse 1,000 ml of dextrose 5% in lactated Ringer's solution over 4 hours." At what rate will this hypertonic solution infuse if the tubing has a drop factor of 10 gtt = 1 ml?

A. 20 gtt/minute
B. 42 gtt/minute
C. 50 gtt/minute
D. 67 gtt/minute

14 The physician orders 200 ml of 0.45% saline solution to be infused in 90 minutes. The drop factor is 10 gtt = 1 ml. What is the correct flow rate for this hypotonic solution?

A. 22 gtt/minute
B. 41 gtt/minute
C. 58 gtt/minute
D. 80 gtt/minute

15 A patient is to receive an infusion of 1,500 ml of D_5W over 16 hours. Available tubing has a drop factor labeled 15 gtt = 1 ml. What is the correct flow rate for this intravenous isotonic solution?

A. 23 gtt/minute
B. 48 gtt/minute
C. 98 gtt/minute
D. 102 gtt/minute

16 An I.V. infusion of 1,000 ml of dextrose 5% in 0.45% saline solution is scheduled to start at 1:30 p.m. and end at 4:30 p.m. The drop factor is 10 gtt = 1 ml. What is the appropriate flow rate?

A. 25 gtt/minute
B. 38 gtt/minute
C. 56 gtt/minute
D. 82 gtt/minute

17 A patient is to receive 1 liter of D_5W, infused at a rate of 100 ml/hour. What would be the flow rate of this isotonic solution if the drop factor is 15 gtt/ml?

A. 25 gtt/minute
B. 32 gtt/minute
C. 77 gtt/minute
D. 80 gtt/minute

18 The physician orders 2,000 ml of D_5W I.V. over 16 hours. The drop factor is 15 gtt = 1 ml. What is the correct flow rate for this intravascular volume expander?

A. 31 gtt/minute
B. 59 gtt/minute
C. 71 gtt/minute
D. 76 gtt/minute

19 The physician orders an infusion of 1,250 ml of a hypotonic 0.3% normal saline solution for 8 hours. If the available tubing has a drop factor of 10 gtt = 1 ml, the nurse should set the flow rate for:

A. 13 gtt/minute
B. 19 gtt/minute
C. 26 gtt/minute
D. 32 gtt/minute

20 Postoperative orders for a patient include 2,400 ml of total volume I.V. therapy to be infused over 24 hours. What is the correct flow rate if the drop factor is 15 gtt = 1 ml?

A. 11 gtt/minute
B. 25 gtt/minute
C. 38 gtt/minute
D. 41 gtt/minute

21 The nurse prepares to administer a stat dose of morphine sulfate to be infused with 30 ml of D_5W over 10 minutes. What would be the correct flow rate if the drop factor is 60 mcgtt = 1 ml?

A. 121 mcgtt/minute
B. 180 mcgtt/minute
C. 190 mcgtt/minute
D. 201 mcgtt/minute

22 To treat a patient's intravascular volume deficit, the physician orders 1,000 ml of lactated Ringer's solution to be infused at 70 gtt/minute. The drop factor is 10 gtt = 1 ml. How many milliliters per hour will be infused?

A. 388 ml/hour
B. 420 ml/hour
C. 500 ml/hour
D. 721 ml/hour

23 Strict intake and output records are being charted for a patient. If the I.V. pump is set at 50 mcgtt/minute and tubing calibration is listed at 60 mcgtt = 1 ml, how many milliliters per minute will this patient receive?

A. 0.8 ml/minute
B. 1.25 ml/minute
C. 44 ml/minute
D. 50 ml/minute

24 A preoperative I.V. infusion of 500 ml of D_5W has been started on a 25-year-old patient. Nurse's notes indicate the infusion is running at 15 gtt/minute, and the tubing calibration is 20 gtt = 1 ml. How many milliliters per hour of this isotonic fluid will this patient receive?

A. 29 ml/hour
B. 36 ml/hour
C. 45 ml/hour
D. 88 ml/hour

25 An I.V. infusion of 1,000 ml of dextrose 2.5% in water is started for a 40-year-old patient to aid hydration. The solution is infusing at a rate of 25 gtt/minute with a drop factor of 15 gtt = 1 ml. How many milliliters per hour will this patient receive?

A. 10 ml/hour
B. 25 ml/hour
C. 50 ml/hour
D. 100 ml/hour

26 The nurse begins an infusion of 500 ml of D₅W with penicillin G, with instructions to infuse at a rate of 20 gtt/minute. The drop factor is 10 gtt = 1 ml. How many milliliters of penicillin G solution is this patient receiving every minute?

A. 2 ml/minute
B. 4 ml/minute
C. 7 ml/minute
D. 10 ml/minute

27 Intravenous insulin therapy has been ordered for a patient. The insulin is to be added to 1,000 ml of normal saline solution and infused at a rate of 10 gtt/minute. If the drop factor is 15 gtt = 1 ml, how many milliliters of this hormone preparation will the patient receive every hour?

A. 12 ml/hour
B. 40 ml/hour
C. 64 ml/hour
D. 72 ml/hour

28 The physician orders an I.V. infusion containing oxytocin (Pitocin) with a drop factor of 60 mcgtt = 1 ml and an infusion rate of 100 mcgtt/minute. How many milliliters of this hormone solution will the patient receive every minute?

A. 0.2 ml/minute
B. 0.5 ml/minute
C. 1.3 ml/minute
D. 1.7 ml/minute

29 The physician's order reads "Add 200 units of regular Humulin insulin to 1,000 ml of 0.9% saline solution, to infuse at the rate of 3.6 U per hour." If the drop factor is 60 mcgtt = 1 ml, how many milliliters of this hormone infuse per hour?

A. 1 ml/hour
B. 18 ml/hour
C. 22 ml/hour
D. 70 ml/hour

30 If a patient is receiving a solution of nitroprusside sodium (Nipride) 50 mg in 250 ml of D_5W at a rate of 18 mcgtt/minute, how many milliliters of this vasodilating solution will the patient receive per hour when the drop factor is 60 mcgtt = 1 ml?

A. 18 ml/hour
B. 30 ml/hour
C. 42 ml/hour
D. 50 ml/hour

31 A patient is receiving a solution of 500 ml of D_5W with 500 mg of trimethaphan (Arfonad) at a rate of 1.2 mg/minute. What is the flow rate of this vasodilator, in milliliters per hour, if the drop factor is 15 gtt = 1 ml?

A. 12 ml/hour
B. 29 ml/hour
C. 66.4 ml/hour
D. 72 ml/hour

32 An intravenous infusion of 750 ml is given to a patient at the rate of 35 gtt/minute, with a drop factor of 15 gtt = 1 ml. How many milliliters per minute will the patient receive?

A. 1.3 ml/minute
B. 2.3 ml/minute
C. 4.6 ml/minute
D. 5 ml/minute

33 The nurse has begun infusing 250 ml D_5W with 500 mg of the bronchodilator aminophylline (Aminophyllin) in a patient who is to receive 25 mg/hr by microdrip (60 mcgtt = 1 ml). How many milliliters per hour will be infused?

A. 4.3 ml/hour
B. 12.5 ml/hour
C. 15 ml/hour
D. 40 ml/hour

34 The physician's order reads "Infuse 600 units of heparin every hour." The pharmacy prepares a solution of 250 ml of D_5W containing 12,000 U of heparin. This solution will infuse at how many milliliters per hour?

A. 12.5 ml/hour
B. 30 ml/hour
C. 50 ml/hour
D. 100 ml/hour

35 A patient is receiving isoproterenol (Isuprel) for its antiarrhythmic action. The physician's order reads "Add 2 mg of isoproterenol to 500 ml of D_5W and infuse at 4 mcg/minute." How many milliliters per hour will this patient receive?

A. 10 ml/hour
B. 16 ml/hour
C. 60 ml/hour
D. 100 ml/hour

36 If an I.V. infusing at 50 gtt/minute has 400 ml left in the bag and the drop factor is 20 gtt = 1 ml, for how much longer will the I.V. infuse?

A. 1 hour, 15 minutes
B. 2 hours, 5 minutes
C. 2 hours, 40 minutes
D. 3 hours, 20 minutes

37 At 8 a.m., the nurse notes that a patient's infusion, which is running at 25 gtt/minute, has 250 ml of solution left in the bag. At what time will the infusion end if the drop factor is 10 gtt = 1 ml?

A. 8:25 a.m.
B. 9:01 a.m.
C. 9:15 a.m.
D. 9:40 a.m.

38 At 2 p.m., 300 ml of solution are left in a patient's infusion that flows at 150 mcgtt/minute. If the drop factor is 60 mcgtt = 1 ml, at what time will the infusion end?

A. 4:00 p.m.
B. 4:22 p.m.
C. 5:18 p.m.
D. 6:03 p.m.

39 An infusion of isotonic normal saline solution has been ordered for a 50-year-old patient who may need to undergo surgery. If 500 ml are ordered at a keep-vein-open (KVO) rate of 10 gtt/minute and the drop factor is 15 gtt = 1 ml, how many hours will the infusion last?

A. 6 hours
B. 10 hours
C. 12½ hours
D. 15 hours

40 A postoperative patient has been receiving parenteral fluids (drop factor is 60 mcgtt = 1 ml). If 75 ml remain to be infused and the flow rate is 30 mcgtt/minute, how many more hours are necessary to complete the infusion?

A. 2½ hours
B. 3 hours
C. 4 hours
D. 5¼ hours

41 A patient's postoperative I.V. therapy calls for 1,000 ml of D_5W to be infused at 150 mcgtt/minute. How much time will the infusion require if the tubing is labeled 60 mcgtt = 1 ml?

A. 1 hour, 50 minutes
B. 2 hours, 14 minutes
C. 4 hours, 3 minutes
D. 6 hours, 40 minutes

42 The physician orders 500 ml of D_5W with 1 g of lidocaine (Xylocaine). The drop factor is 15 gtt = 1 ml. Which flow rate is necessary if the patient is to receive 2 mg/minute?

A. 2 gtt/minute
B. 15 gtt/minute
C. 25 gtt/minute
D. 70 gtt/minute

43 The physician orders 500 ml of D_5W with 100 mg of lidocaine (Xylocaine). The drop factor is 60 mcgtt = 1 ml. Which flow rate would ensure that the patient receives 0.3 mg/minute?

A. 20 mcgtt/minute
B. 55 mcgtt/minute
C. 71 mcgtt/minute
D. 90 mcgtt/minute

44 The physician orders 10 U of oxytocin (Pitocin) to be added to 1,000 ml of D₅W. The drop factor is 60 mcgtt = 1 ml. What would be the flow rate, in microdrops, if the patient is to receive 600 mU/hour of this hormone?

A. 60 mcgtt/minute
B. 84 mcgtt/minute
C. 120 mcgtt/minute
D. 139 mcgtt/minute

45 A patient is to receive 1,000 ml of D₅W to which 1 gr of morphine sulfate has been added. The physician's order stipulates that the patient must receive 1 mg of morphine sulfate every 10 minutes. If the drop factor is 20 gtt = 1 ml, which is the correct flow rate?

A. 26 gtt/minute
B. 33 gtt/minute
C. 89 gtt/minute
D. 120 gtt/minute

46 A patient's chart reads "Administer 150 mg ritodrine (Yutopar) in 500 ml Ringer's solution. Monitor carefully to ensure patient receives 0.35 mg/minute." If the drop factor is 20 gtt = 1 ml, at which flow rate should this uterine relaxant infuse?

A. 23 gtt/minute
B. 40 gtt/minute
C. 69 gtt/minute
D. 125 gtt/minute

47 The physician's order reads "To 1,000 ml D₅W, add 5 million U of aqueous penicillin, and administer 500,000 U/hour." The I.V. tubing has a drop factor of 15 gtt = 1 ml. What is the correct flow rate for this antibiotic preparation?

A. 25 gtt/minute
B. 48 gtt/minute
C. 120 gtt/minute
D. 600 gtt/minute

48 The physician orders 10 mg of phenylephrine (Neo-Synephrine) in 500 ml of D_5W for a hypotensive patient. If the drop factor is 10 gtt = 1 ml, which flow rate will ensure that the patient receives a maintenance dose of 0.05 mg/minute?

A. 1 gtt/minute
B. 13 gtt/minute
C. 25 gtt/minute
D. 40 gtt/minute

49 The nurse prepares to administer 500 ml of D_5W with 40 mEq of potassium chloride at 5 mEq/hour. If the drop factor for the tubing is labeled as 60 mcgtt = 1 ml, she should set the flow rate at:

A. 17 mcgtt/minute
B. 28 mcgtt/minute
C. 63 mcgtt/minute
D. 88 mcgtt/minute

50 The physician's order reads "Prednisolone (Delta-Cortef) 30 mg in 500 ml 0.9% saline solution at 2.5 mg/hour." If the drop factor is 20 gtt = 1 ml, what will be the required flow rate for this drug?

A. 12 gtt/minute
B. 14 gtt/minute
C. 22 gtt/minute
D. 25 gtt/minute

51 The physician's order reads "Add 50 mg of ranitidine (Zantac) to 100 ml of D_5W, and infuse at 2.5 mg/minute." If the drop factor is 10 gtt = 1 ml, the nurse should set the flow rate at:

A. 25 gtt/minute
B. 50 gtt/minute
C. 73 gtt/minute
D. 99 gtt/minute

52 The nurse adds 0.5 g of procainamide (Pronestyl), as ordered, to 250 ml of D$_5$W to infuse at a rate of 5 mg/minute via infusion pump. The drop factor is 20 gtt/ml. The infusion pump should be set at which rate to ensure accurate dosage of this antiarrhythmic solution?

A. 5 gtt/minute
B. 18 gtt/minute
C. 23 gtt/minute
D. 50 gtt/minute

53 As an adjunct to a patient's spinal anesthesia, 100 mg of secobarbital (Seconal) is added to 10 ml of sterile water and infused at 50 mg/90 seconds. If the drop factor is 20 gtt = 1 ml, what is the correct flow rate?

A. 67 gtt/minute
B. 80 gtt/minute
C. 100 gtt/minute
D. 117 gtt/minute

54 The nurse prepares to administer 1,500 mg of tetracycline (Tetracyn) that has been added to 1,000 ml of 0.9 saline solution to infuse at 60 mg/hour. If the drop factor is 20 gtt = 1 ml, the flow rate should be set at:

A. 7 gtt/minute
B. 9 gtt/minute
C. 10 gtt/minute
D. 13 gtt/minute

55 The physician orders 15 mg/kg of the antiviral drug vidarabine (Vira-A) I.V. for a neonate weighing 3 kg. The nurse prepares an infusion by adding 45 mg of the drug to 100 ml of D$_5$W. If the infusion rate is 4 mg/hour and the drop factor is 60 mcgtt = 1 ml, what is the correct flow rate in microdrops/minute?

A. 4 mcgtt/minute
B. 9 mcgtt/minute
C. 12 mcgtt/minute
D. 15 mcgtt/minute

56 The nurse adds 250 mg of niacin (vitamin B_1) to 500 ml normal saline solution, as ordered, to infuse at the rate of 2 mg/minute. The drop factor is 15 gtt = 1 ml. What is the correct flow rate?

A. 27 gtt/minute
B. 35 gtt/minute
C. 50 gtt/minute
D. 60 gtt/minute

57 The nurse prepares an infusion of the antibiotic amikacin (Amikin) by adding 500 mg of the drug to 100 ml of dextrose 5% in normal saline solution. The physician's order stipulates that the patient is to receive 6 mg/minute. If the drop factor is 10 gtt = 1 ml, what is the correct flow rate?

A. 8 gtt/minute
B. 12 gtt/minute
C. 17 gtt/minute
D. 21 gtt/minute

58 The nurse follows a physician's order to administer 30 mg/minute of 50 ml of dextrose 5% in ½ normal saline solution, to which 1 g of azlocillin (Azlin) has been added. What will be the flow rate of this extended-spectrum penicillin if the drop factor is 1 ml = 60 mcgtt?

A. 60 mcgtt/minute
B. 90 mcgtt/minute
C. 120 mcgtt/minute
D. 142 mcgtt/minute

59 The physician's order reads "Administer 500 ml of D_5W with 2,000 mg of bretylium (Bretylol) at 3 mg/minute." What will be the flow rate of this antiarrhythmic solution if the drop factor is 20 gtt = 1 ml?

A. 15 gtt/minute
B. 19 gtt/minute
C. 26 gtt/minute
D. 34 gtt/minute

60 The nurse prepares to administer 1,000 mg of the cephalosoporin cefotaxime (Claforan), which has been added to 250 ml of lactated Ringer's solution, at an infusion rate of 250 mg/hour. If the tubing is calibrated at 15 gtt = 1 ml, what is the correct flow rate?

A. 4 gtt/minute
B. 8 gtt/minute
C. 16 gtt/minute
D. 100 gtt/minute

61 Following physician's orders, the nurse adds 10 mg of the skeletal muscle relaxant diazepam (Valium) to 50 ml of D_5W. If the drop factor is listed as 10 gtt = 1 ml and all the fluid is to be given in 5 minutes, what will be the flow rate?

A. 20 gtt/minute
B. 25 gtt/minute
C. 75 gtt/minute
D. 100 gtt/minute

62 The nurse dilutes 10 mg of cisplatin (Platinol), an antineoplastic agent, in 1,000 ml of dextrose 5% in 0.3% saline solution. Physician's orders indicate that this solution is to infuse at a rate of 1.25 mg/hour. If the drop factor is 20 gtt = 1 ml, the nurse should set the flow rate at:

A. 42 gtt/minute
B. 50 gtt/minute
C. 69 gtt/minute
D. 82 gtt/minute

63 The nurse notes that Mr. S., a patient on the unit, is scheduled to receive clindamycin (Cleocin) via I.V. therapy. To prepare the infusion, she adds 1.2 g of the antibiotic to 200 ml of dextrose 5% in water. If the infusion rate is 600 mg/hour and the drop factor is 20 gtt = 1 ml, what is the flow rate in drops per minute?

A. 5 gtt/minute
B. 12 gtt/minute
C. 15 gtt/minute
D. 33 gtt/minute

64 The physician's order reads "Add 10,000 U of heparin to 1,000 ml of D_5W, and infuse at 250 U/hour." The drop factor is 60 mcgtt = 1 ml. What will be the flow rate for this anticoagulant solution?

A. 9 mcgtt/minute
B. 12 mcgtt/minute
C. 15 mcgtt/minute
D. 25 mcgtt/minute

65 If the above order were increased to 400 U/hour, what would be the adjusted flow rate?

A. 18 mcgtt/minute
B. 40 mcgtt/minute
C. 68 mcgtt/minute
D. 72 mcgtt/minute

66 The physician's order stipulates adding 200 mg of dopamine (Intropin) to 1,000 ml of 0.9% saline solution to infuse at 0.35 mg/minute. How many drops per minute will be administered if the drop factor is 15 gtt = 1 ml?

A. 19 gtt/minute
B. 20 gtt/minute
C. 26 gtt/minute
D. 34 gtt/minute

67 The nurse prepares to administer 1 mg of epinephrine (Adrenalin) added to 250 ml D₅W to infuse at a rate of 1 mcg/minute. The I.V. tubing has a drop factor of 60 mcgtt = 1 ml. What will be the flow rate of this adrenergic stimulant?

A. 5 mcgtt/minute
B. 15 mcgtt/minute
C. 120 mcgtt/minute
D. 138 mcgtt/minute

68 Intravenous lidocaine (Xylocaine) therapy is initiated for a patient. The order reads "Add 1 g of lidocaine to 250 ml D₅W, and infuse at 4 mg/minute." The tubing has a drop factor of 20 gtt = 1 ml. What is the flow rate of this antiarrhythmic drug?

A. 20 gtt/minute
B. 39 gtt/minute
C. 81 gtt/minute
D. 120 gtt/minute

69 The nurse adds 120 mg of morphine sulfate, as ordered, to 500 ml of D₅W to be infused at a rate of 0.3 mg/minute. What will be the flow rate for this narcotic if the tubing is labeled as 10 gtt = 1 ml?

A. 8 gtt/minute
B. 10 gtt/minute
C. 13 gtt/minute
D. 22 gtt/minute

70 The physician orders 1 g of thiopental sodium (Pentothal) added to 500 ml D_5W at an infusion rate of 0.12 g/hour. What is the correct flow rate for this barbiturate if the drop factor is 20 gtt = 1 ml?

A. 2 gtt/minute
B. 4 gtt/minute
C. 16 gtt/minute
D. 20 gtt/minute

71 An obstetric patient is ordered to receive 500 ml D_5W to which 2 g of magnesium sulfate has been added. The nurse notes on the patient's chart that she is to receive 0.5 g every hour. What will be the flow rate of this electrolyte modifier if the drop factor is 15 gtt = 1 ml?

A. 31 gtt/minute
B. 64 gtt/minute
C. 69 gtt/minute
D. 88 gtt/minute

72 An I.V. piggyback of cefoxitin sodium (Mefoxin) has been ordered for Mrs. P. The physician's order stipulates that she is to receive 2 g of the antibiotic added to 100 ml of D_5W and infused at a rate of 1 g/hour via microdrop tubing (60 mcgtt = 1 ml). What will be the flow rate?

A. 14 mcgtt/minute
B. 25 mcgtt/minute
C. 50 mcgtt/minute
D. 78 mcgtt/minute

73 The nurse adds 10,000 U of heparin to 1,000 ml of D_5W, as ordered, for a patient who is to receive 500 U/hour. If the drop factor is 20 gtt = 1 ml, what is the correct flow rate?

A. 9 gtt/minute
B. 10 gtt/minute
C. 11 gtt/minute
D. 17 gtt/minute

74 The nurse administers 5,000 mU of oxytocin (Pitocin) added to 500 ml of D_5W and infused at a rate of 10 mU/minute. The drop factor is labeled as 15 gtt = 1 ml. What is the adjusted flow rate in drops per minute?

A. 15 gtt/minute
B. 38 gtt/minute
C. 42 gtt/minute
D. 61 gtt/minute

75 The nurse transcribes a drug order that reads "Add 75 mg of morphine sulfate to 500 ml normal saline and infuse at 15 mg/hour." The tubing has a drop factor of 20 gtt = 1 ml. What is the adjusted flow rate?

A. 15 gtt/minute
B. 33 gtt/minute
C. 80 gtt/minute
D. 119 gtt/minute

76 The physician orders an infusion of naloxone (Narcan) for a patient because of the drug's narcotic antagonist action. The nurse prepares the infusion by adding 2 mg of naloxone to 500 ml of D₅W, and administers the drug at a rate of 0.04 mg/minute. If the drop factor is 10 gtt = 1 ml, what is the corrected flow rate?

A. 29 gtt/minute
B. 31 gtt/minute
C. 60 gtt/minute
D. 100 gtt/minute

77 A patient must receive 1 mg/minute of lidocaine (Xylocaine). If 1,200 mg have been added to 1,000 ml of D₅W and the drop factor is 60 mcgtt = 1 ml, what will be the flow rate of this antiarrhythmic prepared solution?

A. 35 mcgtt/minute
B. 50 mcgtt/minute
C. 60 mcgtt/minute
D. 93 mcgtt/minute

78 The physician prescribes 25,000 U/minute of penicillin I.V. The nurse prepares the infusion by adding 3 million U to 100 ml of normal saline solution. What will be the flow rate if the drop factor is 15 gtt = 1 ml?

A. 13 gtt/minute
B. 29 gtt/minute
C. 30 gtt/minute
D. 39 gtt/minute

79 The physician has ordered 300 mg of cimetidine (Tagamet) in 100 ml of D₅W to infuse at a rate of 15 mg/minute. Given a drop factor of 10 gtt = 1 ml, what is the flow rate for this antiulcer drug?

A. 10 gtt/minute
B. 25 gtt/minute
C. 50 gtt/minute
D. 100 gtt/minute

80 The nurse prepares to administer 250 mg of the inotropic agent dobutamine (Dobutrex) in 1,000 ml of 0.9% saline solution to infuse at 0.22 mg/minute. The drop factor is 15 gtt = 1 ml. What is the adjusted flow rate for this solution?

A. 13 gtt/minute
B. 39 gtt/minute
C. 42 gtt/minute
D. 70 gtt/minute

81 The physician orders a lidocaine (Xylocaine) drip at 2.6 mg/minute for a patient because of the drug's antiarrhythmic action. The nurse prepares the infusion by adding 0.5 g of lidocaine to 250 ml of D_5W. The drop factor is 60 mcgtt = 1 ml. What will be the flow rate?

A. 20 mcgtt/minute
B. 49 mcgtt/minute
C. 78 mcgtt/minute
D. 92 mcgtt/minute

82 The physician orders oxytocin (Pitocin) for a patient at an infusion rate of 12.5 mU/minute. If 10 U have been added to 750 ml of D_5W and the drop factor is 15 gtt = 1 ml, what is the adjusted flow rate?

A. 3 gtt/minute
B. 14 gtt/minute
C. 50 gtt/minute
D. 78 gtt/minute

83 The nurse prepares an electrolyte solution of 25 mEq of potassium chloride added to 250 ml of D_5W, regulated so that the patient receives 7.5 mEq/hour. The drop factor is 60 mcgtt = 1 ml. What is the adjusted flow rate?

A. 37 mcgtt/minute
B. 41 mcgtt/minute
C. 75 mcgtt/minute
D. 92 mcgtt/minute

84 The physician's order reads "Add 250 mg of dobutamine (Dobutrex) to 250 ml of D_5W to infuse at a rate of 0.005 mg/kg/minute." If the patient weighs 50 kg and the drop factor is 60 mcgtt = 1 ml, what will be the flow rate for this inotropic agent?

A. 15 mcgtt/minute
B. 27 mcgtt/minute
C. 50 mcgtt/minute
D. 55 mcgtt/minute

85 A patient weighing 72 kg needs an infusion of 500 ml D_5W with 400 mg of dopamine (Intropin). The drop factor is 60 mcgtt = 1 ml. What is the flow rate if the patient is to receive 0.01 mg/kg/minute of this vasopressor drug?

A. 14 mcgtt/minute
B. 54 mcgtt/minute
C. 80 mcgtt/minute
D. 142 mcgtt/minute

86 The nurse prepares a continuous infusion of the bronchodilator aminophylline (Aminophyllin) for a patient weighing 65 kg. The physician's order reads "Add 350 mg aminophylline to 500 ml of D_5W, and give 0.008 mg/kg/minute." What will be the flow rate if the tubing has a drop factor of 60 mcgtt = 1 ml?

A. 19 mcgtt/minute
B. 24 mcgtt/minute
C. 45 mcgtt/minute
D. 91 mcgtt/minute

87 The physician orders I.V. urokinase (Abbokinase) 4,400 I.U./kg/hour for a 50-kg patient with deep vein thrombosis. The nurse adds 2.5 million U of urokinase to 1,000 ml of D_5W, and notes that the drop factor is listed as 15 gtt = 1 ml. What is the adjusted flow rate for this infusion?

A. 6 gtt/minute
B. 12 gtt/minute
C. 22 gtt/minute
D. 40 gtt/minute

88 The physician orders a solution of 250 ml D_5W with 50 mg of nitroprusside sodium (Nipride) to infuse at the rate of 0.5 mcg/kg/minute. The patient weighs 70 kg. What would be the flow rate for this vasodilator if the drop factor were 60 mcgtt = 1 ml?

A. 11 mcgtt/minute
B. 45 mcgtt/minute
C. 80 mcgtt/minute
D. 128 mcgtt/minute

Answer sheet

	A B C D		A B C D		A B C D
1	○ ○ ○ ○	31	○ ○ ○ ○	61	○ ○ ○ ○
2	○ ○ ○ ○	32	○ ○ ○ ○	62	○ ○ ○ ○
3	○ ○ ○ ○	33	○ ○ ○ ○	63	○ ○ ○ ○
4	○ ○ ○ ○	34	○ ○ ○ ○	64	○ ○ ○ ○
5	○ ○ ○ ○	35	○ ○ ○ ○	65	○ ○ ○ ○
6	○ ○ ○ ○	36	○ ○ ○ ○	66	○ ○ ○ ○
7	○ ○ ○ ○	37	○ ○ ○ ○	67	○ ○ ○ ○
8	○ ○ ○ ○	38	○ ○ ○ ○	68	○ ○ ○ ○
9	○ ○ ○ ○	39	○ ○ ○ ○	69	○ ○ ○ ○
10	○ ○ ○ ○	40	○ ○ ○ ○	70	○ ○ ○ ○
11	○ ○ ○ ○	41	○ ○ ○ ○	71	○ ○ ○ ○
12	○ ○ ○ ○	42	○ ○ ○ ○	72	○ ○ ○ ○
13	○ ○ ○ ○	43	○ ○ ○ ○	73	○ ○ ○ ○
14	○ ○ ○ ○	44	○ ○ ○ ○	74	○ ○ ○ ○
15	○ ○ ○ ○	45	○ ○ ○ ○	75	○ ○ ○ ○
16	○ ○ ○ ○	46	○ ○ ○ ○	76	○ ○ ○ ○
17	○ ○ ○ ○	47	○ ○ ○ ○	77	○ ○ ○ ○
18	○ ○ ○ ○	48	○ ○ ○ ○	78	○ ○ ○ ○
19	○ ○ ○ ○	49	○ ○ ○ ○	79	○ ○ ○ ○
20	○ ○ ○ ○	50	○ ○ ○ ○	80	○ ○ ○ ○
21	○ ○ ○ ○	51	○ ○ ○ ○	81	○ ○ ○ ○
22	○ ○ ○ ○	52	○ ○ ○ ○	82	○ ○ ○ ○
23	○ ○ ○ ○	53	○ ○ ○ ○	83	○ ○ ○ ○
24	○ ○ ○ ○	54	○ ○ ○ ○	84	○ ○ ○ ○
25	○ ○ ○ ○	55	○ ○ ○ ○	85	○ ○ ○ ○
26	○ ○ ○ ○	56	○ ○ ○ ○	86	○ ○ ○ ○
27	○ ○ ○ ○	57	○ ○ ○ ○	87	○ ○ ○ ○
28	○ ○ ○ ○	58	○ ○ ○ ○	88	○ ○ ○ ○
29	○ ○ ○ ○	59	○ ○ ○ ○		
30	○ ○ ○ ○	60	○ ○ ○ ○		

Answers

1 Correct answer—**B**

D/A

$$\frac{1,500 \text{ ml}}{12 \text{ hr}} \times \frac{\overset{1}{\cancel{15}} \text{ gtt}}{1 \text{ ml}} \times \frac{1 \text{ hr}}{\underset{4}{\cancel{60}} \text{ min}} = \frac{1,500 \text{ gtt}}{48 \text{ min}} = 31.2 \text{ or } 31 \text{ gtt/minute}$$

R/P

Step 1: Change milliliters to drops.

$$1 \text{ ml} : 15 \text{ gtt} :: 1,500 \text{ ml} : x \text{ gtt}$$
$$x = 15 \times 1,500$$
$$x = 22,500 \text{ gtt}$$

Step 2: Change hours to minutes.

$$1 \text{ hr} : 60 \text{ min} :: 12 \text{ hr} : x \text{ min}$$
$$x = 60 \times 12$$
$$x = 720 \text{ minutes}$$

Step 3: Calculate the flow rate.

$$720 \text{ min} : 22,500 \text{ gtt} :: 1 \text{ min} : x \text{ gtt}$$
$$720x = 22,500$$
$$x = \frac{22,500}{720}$$
$$x = 31.2 \text{ or } 31 \text{ gtt/minute}$$

2 Correct answer—**A**

D/A

$$\frac{1,000 \text{ ml}}{24 \text{ hr}} \times \frac{\overset{1}{\cancel{60}} \text{ mcgtt}}{1 \text{ ml}} \times \frac{1 \text{ hr}}{\underset{1}{\cancel{60}} \text{ min}} =$$

$$\frac{1,000 \text{ mcgtt}}{24 \text{ min}} = 41.6 \text{ or } 42 \text{ mcgtt/minute}$$

R/P

Step 1: Change milliliters to microdrops.

$$1 \text{ ml} : 60 \text{ mcgtt} :: 1,000 \text{ ml} : x \text{ mcgtt}$$
$$x = 60 \times 1,000$$
$$x = 60,000 \text{ mcgtt}$$

Step 2: Change hours to minutes.

$$1 \text{ hr} : 60 \text{ min} :: 24 \text{ hr} : x \text{ min}$$
$$x = 60 \times 24$$
$$x = 1,440 \text{ minutes}$$

Step 3: Calculate the flow rate.

1,440 min : 60,000 mcgtt :: 1 min : x mcgtt

$$1,440x = 60,000$$

$$x = \frac{60,000}{1,440}$$

$$x = 41.6 \text{ or } 42 \text{ mcgtt/minute}$$

---

3 Correct answer — **C**

D/A

$$\frac{\overset{5}{\cancel{150} \text{ ml}}}{\underset{1}{\cancel{30} \text{ min}}} \times \frac{10 \text{ gtt}}{1 \text{ ml}} = 50 \text{ gtt/minute}$$

R/P

Step 1: Change milliliters to drops.

1 ml : 10 gtt :: 150 ml : x gtt

$$x = 10 \times 150$$

$$x = 1,500 \text{ gtt}$$

Step 2: Calculate the flow rate.

30 min : 1,500 gtt :: 1 min : x gtt

$$30x = 1,500$$

$$x = \frac{1,500}{30}$$

$$x = 50 \text{ gtt/minute}$$

---

4 Correct answer — **D**

D/A

$$\frac{500 \text{ ml}}{4 \text{ hr}} \times \frac{\overset{1}{\cancel{20} \text{ gtt}}}{1 \text{ ml}} \times \frac{1 \text{ hr}}{\underset{3}{\cancel{60} \text{ min}}} = \frac{500 \text{ gtt}}{12 \text{ min}} = 41.6 \text{ or } 42 \text{ gtt/minute}$$

R/P

Step 1: Change milliliters to drops.

1 ml : 20 gtt :: 500 ml : x gtt

$$x = 20 \times 500$$

$$x = 10,000 \text{ gtt}$$

Step 2: Change hours to minutes.

1 hr : 60 min :: 4 hr : x min

$$x = 60 \times 4$$

$$x = 240 \text{ minutes}$$

Step 3: Calculate the flow rate.

$$240 \text{ min} : 10{,}000 \text{ gtt} :: 1 \text{ min} : x \text{ gtt}$$
$$240x = 10{,}000$$
$$x = \frac{10{,}000}{240}$$
$$x = 41.6 \text{ or } 42 \text{ gtt/minute}$$

5 Correct answer — **C**

D/A

$$\frac{125 \cancel{\text{ml}}^{\,} }{\underset{3}{\cancel{90}} \text{ min}} \times \frac{\overset{2}{\cancel{60}} \text{ mcgtt}}{1 \cancel{\text{ml}}} = \frac{250 \text{ mcgtt}}{3 \text{ min}} = 83.3 \text{ or } 83 \text{ mcgtt/minute}$$

R/P

Step 1: Change milliliters to microdrops.

$$1 \text{ ml} : 60 \text{ mcgtt} :: 125 \text{ ml} : x \text{ mcgtt}$$
$$x = 60 \times 125$$
$$x = 7{,}500 \text{ mcgtt}$$

Step 2: Calculate the flow rate.

$$90 \text{ min} : 7{,}500 \text{ mcgtt} :: 1 \text{ min} : x \text{ mcgtt}$$
$$90x = 7{,}500$$
$$x = \frac{7{,}500}{90}$$
$$x = 83.3 \text{ or } 83 \text{ mcgtt/minute}$$

6 Correct answer — **A**

D/A

$$\frac{2{,}500 \cancel{\text{ml}}}{24 \cancel{\text{hr}}} \times \frac{\overset{1}{\cancel{10}} \text{ gtt}}{1 \cancel{\text{ml}}} \times \frac{1 \cancel{\text{hr}}}{\underset{6}{\cancel{60}} \text{ min}} = \frac{2{,}500 \text{ gtt}}{144 \text{ min}} = 17.3 \text{ or } 17 \text{ gtt/minute}$$

R/P

Step 1: Change milliliters to drops.

$$1 \text{ ml} : 10 \text{ gtt} :: 2{,}500 \text{ ml} : x \text{ gtt}$$
$$x = 10 \times 2{,}500$$
$$x = 25{,}000 \text{ gtt}$$

Step 2: Change hours to minutes.

$$1 \text{ hr} : 60 \text{ min} :: 24 \text{ hr} : x \text{ min}$$
$$x = 60 \times 24$$
$$x = 1{,}440 \text{ minutes}$$

Step 3: Calculate the flow rate.

$$1{,}440 \text{ min} : 25{,}000 \text{ gtt} :: 1 \text{ min} : x \text{ gtt}$$
$$1{,}440x = 25{,}000$$
$$x = \frac{25{,}000}{1{,}440}$$
$$x = 17.3 \text{ or } 17 \text{ gtt/minute}$$

7 Correct answer — **B**

D/A

$$\frac{3{,}000 \ \cancel{ml}}{24 \ \cancel{hr}} \times \frac{\overset{1}{\cancel{10}} \text{ gtt}}{1 \ \cancel{ml}} \times \frac{1 \ \cancel{hr}}{\underset{6}{\cancel{60}} \text{ min}} = \frac{3{,}000 \text{ gtt}}{144 \text{ min}} = 20.8 \text{ or } 21 \text{ gtt/minute}$$

R/P

Step 1: Change milliliters to drops.

$$1 \text{ ml} : 10 \text{ gtt} :: 3{,}000 \text{ ml} : x \text{ gtt}$$
$$x = 10 \times 3{,}000$$
$$x = 30{,}000 \text{ gtt}$$

Step 2: Change hours to minutes.

$$1 \text{ hr} : 60 \text{ min} :: 24 \text{ hr} : x \text{ min}$$
$$x = 60 \times 24$$
$$x = 1{,}440 \text{ minutes}$$

Step 3: Calculate the flow rate.

$$1{,}440 \text{ min} : 30{,}000 \text{ gtt} :: 1 \text{ min} : x \text{ gtt}$$
$$1{,}440x = 30{,}000$$
$$x = \frac{30{,}000}{1{,}440}$$
$$x = 20.8 \text{ or } 21 \text{ gtt/minute}$$

8 Correct answer — **A**

D/A

$$\frac{750 \ \cancel{ml}}{8 \ \cancel{hr}} \times \frac{\overset{1}{\cancel{15}} \text{ gtt}}{1 \ \cancel{ml}} \times \frac{1 \ \cancel{hr}}{\underset{4}{\cancel{60}} \text{ min}} = \frac{750 \text{ gtt}}{32 \text{ min}} = 23.4 \text{ or } 23 \text{ gtt/minute}$$

R/P

Step 1: Change milliliters to drops.

$$1 \text{ ml} : 15 \text{ gtt} :: 750 \text{ ml} : x \text{ gtt}$$
$$x = 15 \times 750$$
$$x = 11{,}250 \text{ gtt}$$

Step 2: Change hours to minutes.

$$1 \text{ hr} : 60 \text{ min} :: 8 \text{ hr} : x \text{ min}$$
$$x = 60 \times 8$$
$$x = 480 \text{ minutes}$$

Step 3: Calculate the flow rate.

$$480 \text{ min} : 11{,}250 \text{ gtt} :: 1 \text{ min} : x \text{ gtt}$$
$$480x = 11{,}250$$
$$x = \frac{11{,}250}{480}$$
$$x = 23.4 \text{ or } 23 \text{ gtt/minute}$$

9 Correct answer — B

D/A

$$\frac{400 \text{ ml}}{4 \text{ hr}} \times \frac{\overset{1}{\cancel{60}} \text{ mcgtt}}{1 \text{ ml}} \times \frac{1 \text{ hr}}{\underset{1}{\cancel{60}} \text{ min}} = \frac{400 \text{ mcgtt}}{4 \text{ min}} = 100 \text{ mcgtt/minute}$$

R/P

Step 1: Change milliliters to microdrops.

$$1 \text{ ml} : 60 \text{ mcgtt} :: 400 \text{ ml} : x \text{ mcgtt}$$
$$x = 60 \times 400$$
$$x = 24{,}000 \text{ mcgtt}$$

Step 2: Change hours to minutes.

$$1 \text{ hr} : 60 \text{ min} :: 4 \text{ hr} : x \text{ min}$$
$$x = 60 \times 4$$
$$x = 240 \text{ minutes}$$

Step 3: Calculate the flow rate.

$$240 \text{ min} : 24{,}000 \text{ mcgtt} :: 1 \text{ min} : x \text{ mcgtt}$$
$$240x = 24{,}000$$
$$x = \frac{24{,}000}{240}$$
$$x = 100 \text{ mcgtt/minute}$$

10 Correct answer — D

D/A

$$\frac{1{,}000 \text{ ml}}{6 \text{ hr}} \times \frac{\overset{1}{\cancel{10}} \text{ gtt}}{1 \text{ ml}} \times \frac{1 \text{ hr}}{\underset{6}{\cancel{60}} \text{ min}} = \frac{1{,}000 \text{ gtt}}{36 \text{ min}} = 27.7 \text{ or } 28 \text{ gtt/minute}$$

R/P

Step 1: Change milliliters to drops.
$$1 \text{ ml} : 10 \text{ gtt} :: 1,000 \text{ ml} : x \text{ gtt}$$
$$x = 10 \times 1,000$$
$$x = 10,000 \text{ gtt}$$

Step 2: Change hours to minutes.
$$1 \text{ hr} : 60 \text{ min} :: 6 \text{ hr} : x \text{ min}$$
$$x = 60 \times 6$$
$$x = 360 \text{ minutes}$$

Step 3: Calculate the flow rate.

$$360 \text{ min} : 10,000 \text{ gtt} :: 1 \text{ min} : x \text{ gtt}$$
$$360x = 10,000$$
$$x = \frac{10,000}{360}$$
$$x = 27.7 \text{ or } 28 \text{ gtt/minute}$$

11 Correct answer — **D**

D/A

$$\frac{500 \ \cancel{ml}}{2 \ \cancel{hr}} \times \frac{\overset{1}{\cancel{10}} \text{ gtt}}{1 \ \cancel{ml}} \times \frac{1 \ \cancel{hr}}{\underset{6}{\cancel{60}} \text{ min}} = \frac{500 \text{ gtt}}{12 \text{ min}} = 41.6 \text{ or } 42 \text{ gtt/minute}$$

R/P

Step 1: Change milliliters to drops.
$$1 \text{ ml} : 10 \text{ gtt} :: 500 \text{ ml} : x \text{ gtt}$$
$$x = 10 \times 500$$
$$x = 5,000 \text{ gtt}$$

Step 2: Change hours to minutes.
$$1 \text{ hr} : 60 \text{ min} :: 2 \text{ hr} : x \text{ min}$$
$$x = 60 \times 2$$
$$x = 120 \text{ minutes}$$

Step 3: Calculate the flow rate.
$$120 \text{ min} : 5,000 \text{ gtt} :: 1 \text{ min} : x \text{ gtt}$$
$$120x = 5,000$$
$$x = \frac{5,000}{120}$$
$$x = 41.6 \text{ or } 42 \text{ gtt/minute}$$

12 Correct answer — **A**

D/A

$$\frac{\overset{1}{\cancel{100}} \ \cancel{ml}}{\underset{1}{\cancel{60}} \ min} \times \frac{\overset{1}{\cancel{60}} \ mcgtt}{1 \ \cancel{ml}} = 100 \ mcgtt/minute$$

R/P

Step 1: Change milliliters to microdrops.

1 ml : 60 mcgtt :: 100 ml : x mcgtt

$x = 60 \times 100$

$x = 6,000$ mcgtt

Step 2: Calculate the flow rate.

60 min : 6,000 mcgtt :: 1 min : x mcgtt

$60x = 6,000$

$x = \dfrac{6,000}{60}$

$x = 100$ mcgtt/minute

13 Correct answer — **B**

D/A

$$\frac{1,000 \ \cancel{ml}}{4 \ \cancel{hr}} \times \frac{\overset{1}{\cancel{10}} \ gtt}{1 \ \cancel{ml}} \times \frac{1 \ \cancel{hr}}{\underset{6}{\cancel{60}} \ min} = \frac{1,000 \ gtt}{24 \ min} = 41.6 \ or \ 42 \ gtt/minute$$

R/P

Step 1: Change milliliters to drops.

1 ml : 10 gtt :: 1,000 ml : x gtt

$x = 10 \times 1,000$

$x = 10,000$ gtt

Step 2: Change hours to minutes.

1 hr : 60 min :: 4 hr : x min

$x = 60 \times 4$

$x = 240$ minutes

Step 3: Calculate the flow rate.

240 min : 10,000 gtt :: 1 min : x gtt

$240x = 10,000$

$x = \dfrac{10,000}{240}$

$x = 41.6$ or 42 gtt/minute

14 Correct answer — **A**

D/A

$$\frac{200 \text{ ml}}{\underset{9}{90} \text{ min}} \times \frac{\overset{1}{10} \text{ gtt}}{1 \text{ ml}} = \frac{200 \text{ gtt}}{9 \text{ min}} = 22.2 \text{ or } 22 \text{ gtt/minute}$$

R/P

Step 1: Change milliliters to drops.

1 ml : 10 gtt :: 200 ml : x gtt
$x = 10 \times 200$
$x = 2,000$ gtt

Step 2: Calculate the flow rate.

90 min : 2,000 gtt :: 1 min : x gtt
$90x = 2,000$
$x = \dfrac{2,000}{90}$
$x = 22.2$ or 22 gtt/minute

15 Correct answer — **A**

D/A

$$\frac{1,500 \text{ ml}}{16 \text{ hr}} \times \frac{\overset{1}{15} \text{ gtt}}{1 \text{ ml}} \times \frac{1 \text{ hr}}{\underset{4}{60} \text{ min}} = \frac{1,500 \text{ gtt}}{64 \text{ min}} = 23.4 \text{ or } 23 \text{ gtt/minute}$$

R/P

Step 1: Change milliliters to drops.

1 ml : 15 gtt :: 1,500 ml : x gtt
$x = 15 \times 1,500$
$x = 22,500$ gtt

Step 2: Change hours to minutes.

1 hr : 60 min :: 16 hr : x min
$x = 60 \times 16$
$x = 960$ minutes

Step 3: Calculate the flow rate.

960 min : 22,500 gtt :: 1 min : x gtt
$960x = 22,500$
$x = \dfrac{22,500}{960}$
$x = 23.4$ or 23 gtt/minute

16 Correct answer — C

D/A

$$\frac{1,000 \text{ ml}}{3 \text{ hr}} \times \frac{\overset{1}{\cancel{10}} \text{ gtt}}{1 \text{ ml}} \times \frac{1 \text{ hr}}{\underset{6}{\cancel{60}} \text{ min}} = \frac{1,000 \text{ gtt}}{18 \text{ min}} = 55.5 \text{ or } 56 \text{ gtt/minute}$$

R/P

Step 1: Change milliliters to drops.

$$1 \text{ ml} : 10 \text{ gtt} :: 1,000 \text{ ml} : x \text{ gtt}$$
$$x = 10 \times 1,000$$
$$x = 10,000 \text{ gtt}$$

Step 2: Change hours to minutes.

$$1 \text{ hr} : 60 \text{ min} :: 3 \text{ hr} : x \text{ min}$$
$$x = 60 \times 3$$
$$x = 180 \text{ minutes}$$

Step 3: Calculate the flow rate.

$$180 \text{ min} : 10,000 \text{ gtt} :: 1 \text{ min} : x \text{ gtt}$$
$$180x = 10,000$$
$$x = \frac{10,000}{180}$$
$$x = 55.5 \text{ or } 56 \text{ gtt/minute}$$

17 Correct answer — A

D/A

$$\frac{100 \text{ ml}}{\underset{4}{\cancel{60}} \text{ min}} \times \frac{\overset{1}{\cancel{15}} \text{ gtt}}{1 \text{ ml}} = \frac{100 \text{ gtt}}{4 \text{ min}} = 25 \text{ gtt/minute}$$

R/P

Step 1: Change milliliters to drops.

$$1 \text{ ml} : 15 \text{ gtt} :: 100 \text{ ml} : x \text{ gtt}$$
$$x = 15 \times 100$$
$$x = 1,500 \text{ gtt}$$

Step 2: Calculate flow rate.

$$60 \text{ min} : 1,500 \text{ gtt} :: 1 \text{ min} : x \text{ gtt}$$
$$60x = 1,500$$
$$x = \frac{1,500}{60}$$
$$x = 25 \text{ gtt/minute}$$

18 Correct answer — **A**

D/A

$$\frac{2,000 \text{ ml}}{16 \text{ hr}} \times \frac{\overset{1}{\cancel{15}} \text{ gtt}}{1 \text{ ml}} \times \frac{1 \text{ hr}}{\underset{4}{\cancel{60}} \text{ min}} = \frac{2,000 \text{ gtt}}{64 \text{ min}} = 31.2 \text{ or } 31 \text{ gtt/minute}$$

R/P

Step 1: Change milliliters to drops.

$$1 \text{ ml} : 15 \text{ gtt} :: 2,000 \text{ ml} : x \text{ gtt}$$
$$x = 15 \times 2,000$$
$$x = 30,000 \text{ gtt}$$

Step 2: Change hours to minutes.

$$1 \text{ hr} : 60 \text{ min} :: 16 \text{ hr} : x \text{ min}$$
$$x = 60 \times 16$$
$$x = 960 \text{ minutes}$$

Step 3: Calculate the flow rate.

$$960 \text{ min} : 30,000 \text{ gtt} :: 1 \text{ min} : x \text{ gtt}$$
$$960x = 30,000$$
$$x = \frac{30,000}{960}$$
$$x = 31.2 \text{ or } 31 \text{ gtt/minute}$$

19 Correct answer — **C**

D/A

$$\frac{1,250 \text{ ml}}{8 \text{ hr}} \times \frac{\overset{1}{\cancel{10}} \text{ gtt}}{1 \text{ ml}} \times \frac{1 \text{ hr}}{\underset{6}{\cancel{60}} \text{ min}} = \frac{1,250 \text{ gtt}}{48 \text{ min}} = 26 \text{ gtt/minute}$$

R/P

Step 1: Change milliliters to drops.

$$1 \text{ ml} : 10 \text{ gtt} :: 1,250 \text{ ml} : x \text{ gtt}$$
$$x = 10 \times 1,250$$
$$x = 12,500 \text{ gtt}$$

Step 2: Change hours to minutes.

$$1 \text{ hr} : 60 \text{ min} :: 8 \text{ hr} : x \text{ min}$$
$$x = 60 \times 8$$
$$x = 480 \text{ minutes}$$

Step 3: Calculate the flow rate.

$$480 \text{ min} : 12,500 \text{ gtt} :: 1 \text{ min} : x \text{ gtt}$$
$$480x = 12,500$$
$$x = \frac{12,500}{480}$$
$$x = 26 \text{ gtt/minute}$$

20 Correct answer — **B**

D/A

$$\frac{\overset{100}{\cancel{2,400}} \cancel{\text{ml}}}{\underset{1}{\cancel{24} \cancel{\text{hr}}}} \times \frac{\overset{1}{\cancel{15}} \text{gtt}}{1 \cancel{\text{ml}}} \times \frac{1 \cancel{\text{hr}}}{\underset{4}{\cancel{60}} \text{min}} = \frac{100 \text{ gtt}}{4 \text{ min}} = 25 \text{ gtt/minute}$$

R/P

Step 1: Change milliliters to drops.

$$1 \text{ ml} : 15 \text{ gtt} :: 2,400 \text{ ml} : x \text{ gtt}$$
$$x = 15 \times 2,400$$
$$x = 36,000 \text{ gtt}$$

Step 2: Change hours to minutes.

$$1 \text{ hr} : 60 \text{ min} :: 24 \text{ hr} : x \text{ min}$$
$$x = 60 \times 24$$
$$x = 1,440 \text{ minutes}$$

Step 3: Calculate the flow rate.

$$1,440 \text{ min} : 36,000 \text{ gtt} :: 1 \text{ min} : x \text{ gtt}$$
$$1,440x = 36,000$$
$$x = \frac{36,000}{1,440}$$
$$x = 25 \text{ gtt/minute}$$

21 Correct answer — **B**

D/A

$$\frac{30 \cancel{\text{ml}}}{\underset{1}{\cancel{10}} \text{min}} \times \frac{\overset{6}{\cancel{60}} \text{mcgtt}}{1 \cancel{\text{ml}}} = 180 \text{ mcgtt/minute}$$

R/P

Step 1: Change milliliters to microdrops.

$$1 \text{ ml} : 60 \text{ mcgtt} :: 30 \text{ ml} : x \text{ mcgtt}$$
$$x = 60 \times 30$$
$$x = 1,800 \text{ mcgtt}$$

Step 2: Calculate the flow rate.

$$10 \text{ min} : 1,800 \text{ mcgtt} :: 1 \text{ min} : x \text{ mcgtt}$$
$$10x = 1,800$$
$$x = \frac{1,800}{10}$$
$$x = 180 \text{ mcgtt/minute}$$

22 Correct answer — B

D/A

$$\frac{70 \text{ gtt}}{1 \text{ min}} \times \frac{1 \text{ ml}}{\overset{}{\underset{1}{10}} \text{ gtt}} \times \frac{\overset{6}{60} \text{ min}}{1 \text{ hr}} = 420 \text{ ml/hour}$$

R/P

Step 1: Change drops to milliliters.

$$10 \text{ gtt} : 1 \text{ ml} :: 70 \text{ gtt} : x \text{ ml}$$
$$10x = 70$$
$$x = \frac{70}{10}$$
$$x = 7 \text{ ml}$$

Step 2: Calculate the number of milliliters per hour.

$$1 \text{ min} : 7 \text{ ml} :: 60 \text{ min} : x \text{ ml}$$
$$x = 7 \times 60$$
$$x = 420 \text{ ml/hour}$$

23 Correct answer — A

D/A

$$\frac{\overset{5}{50} \text{ mcgtt}}{1 \text{ min}} \times \frac{1 \text{ ml}}{\underset{6}{60} \text{ mcgtt}} = \frac{5 \text{ ml}}{6 \text{ min}} = 0.83 \text{ or } 0.8 \text{ ml/minute}$$

R/P

$$60 \text{ mcgtt} : 1 \text{ ml} :: 50 \text{ mcgtt} : x \text{ ml}$$
$$60x = 50$$
$$x = \frac{50}{60}$$
$$x = 0.83 \text{ or } 0.8 \text{ ml/minute}$$

24 Correct answer — C

D/A

$$\frac{15 \text{ gtt}}{1 \text{ min}} \times \frac{1 \text{ ml}}{\underset{1}{\cancel{20} \text{ gtt}}} \times \frac{\overset{3}{\cancel{60} \text{ min}}}{1 \text{ hr}} = 45 \text{ ml/hour}$$

R/P

Step 1: Change drops to milliliters.

$$20 \text{ gtt} : 1 \text{ ml} :: 15 \text{ gtt} : x \text{ ml}$$
$$20x = 15$$
$$x = \frac{15}{20}$$
$$x = 0.75 \text{ ml}$$

Step 2: Calculate the number of milliliters per hour.

$$1 \text{ min} : 0.75 \text{ ml} :: 60 \text{ min} : x \text{ ml}$$
$$x = 0.75 \times 60$$
$$x = 45 \text{ ml/hour}$$

25 Correct answer — D

D/A

$$\frac{25 \text{ gtt}}{1 \text{ min}} \times \frac{1 \text{ ml}}{\underset{1}{\cancel{15} \text{ gtt}}} \times \frac{\overset{4}{\cancel{60} \text{ min}}}{1 \text{ hr}} = 100 \text{ ml/hour}$$

R/P

Step 1: Change drops to milliliters.

$$15 \text{ gtt} : 1 \text{ ml} :: 25 \text{ gtt} : x \text{ ml}$$
$$15x = 25$$
$$x = \frac{25}{15}$$
$$x = 1.66 \text{ ml}$$

Step 2: Calculate the number of milliliters per hour.

$$1 \text{ min} : 1.66 \text{ ml} :: 60 \text{ min} : x \text{ ml}$$
$$x = 1.66 \times 60$$
$$x = 99.9 \text{ or } 100 \text{ ml/hour}$$

26 Correct answer — **A**

D/A

$$\frac{\overset{2}{\cancel{20} \text{ gtt}}}{1 \text{ min}} \times \frac{1 \text{ ml}}{\underset{1}{\cancel{10} \text{ gtt}}} = 2 \text{ ml/minute}$$

R/P

$$10 \text{ gtt} : 1 \text{ ml} :: 20 \text{ gtt} : x \text{ ml}$$
$$10x = 20$$
$$x = \frac{20}{10}$$
$$x = 2 \text{ ml/minute}$$

27 Correct answer — **B**

D/A

$$\frac{10 \text{ gtt}}{1 \text{ min}} \times \frac{1 \text{ ml}}{\underset{1}{\cancel{15} \text{ gtt}}} \times \frac{\overset{4}{\cancel{60} \text{ min}}}{1 \text{ hr}} = 40 \text{ ml/hour}$$

R/P

Step 1: Change drops to milliliters.
$$15 \text{ gtt} : 1 \text{ ml} :: 10 \text{ gtt} : x \text{ ml}$$
$$15x = 10$$
$$x = \frac{10}{15}$$
$$x = 0.66 \text{ ml}$$

Step 2: Calculate the number of milliliters per hour.
$$1 \text{ min} : 0.66 \text{ ml} :: 60 \text{ min} : x \text{ ml}$$
$$x = 0.66 \times 60$$
$$x = 39.6 \text{ or } 40 \text{ ml/hour}$$

28 Correct answer — **D**

D/A
$$\frac{\cancel{100} \text{ mcgtt}}{1 \text{ min}} \times \frac{1 \text{ ml}}{\cancel{60} \text{ mcgtt}} = \frac{10 \text{ ml}}{6 \text{ min}} = 1.66 \text{ or } 1.7 \text{ ml/minute}$$

R/P
$$60 \text{ mcgtt} : 1 \text{ ml} :: 100 \text{ mcgtt} : x \text{ ml}$$
$$60x = 100$$
$$x = \frac{100}{60}$$
$$x = 1.66 \text{ or } 1.7 \text{ ml/minute}$$

29 Correct answer—**B**

D/A

$$\frac{3.6 \cancel{U}}{1 \text{ hr}} \times \frac{\overset{5}{\cancel{1,000}} \text{ ml}}{\underset{1}{\cancel{200}} \cancel{U}} = 18 \text{ ml/hour}$$

R/P

$$200 \text{ U} : 1,000 \text{ ml} :: 3.6 \text{ U} : x \text{ ml}$$
$$200x = 1,000 \times 3.6$$
$$x = \frac{3,600}{200}$$
$$x = 18 \text{ ml/hour}$$

30 Correct answer—**A**

Remember: microdrops per minute equal milliliters per hour.
$$18 \text{ mcgtt/minute} = 18 \text{ ml/hour}$$

D/A

$$\frac{18 \text{ mcgtt}}{1 \text{ min}} \times \frac{1 \text{ ml}}{\underset{1}{\cancel{60}} \text{ mcgtt}} \times \frac{\overset{1}{\cancel{60}} \text{ min}}{1 \text{ hr}} = 18 \text{ ml/hour}$$

R/P

Step 1: Change microdrops to milliliters.
$$60 \text{ mcgtt} : 1 \text{ ml} :: 18 \text{ mcgtt} : x \text{ ml}$$
$$60x = 18$$
$$x = \frac{18}{60}$$
$$x = 0.3 \text{ ml}$$

Step 2: Calculate the number of milliliters per hour.
$$1 \text{ min} : 0.3 \text{ ml} :: 60 \text{ min} : x \text{ ml}$$
$$x = 0.3 \times 60$$
$$x = 18 \text{ ml/hour}$$

31 Correct answer—**D**

D/A

$$\frac{1.2 \cancel{mg}}{1 \text{ min}} \times \frac{\overset{1}{\cancel{500}} \text{ ml}}{\underset{1}{\cancel{500}} \cancel{mg}} \times \frac{60 \text{ min}}{1 \text{ hr}} = 72 \text{ ml/hour}$$

R/P

Step 1: Calculate required milliliters.
$$500 \text{ mg} : 500 \text{ ml} :: 1.2 \text{ mg} : x \text{ ml}$$
$$x = 1.2 \text{ ml}$$

Step 2: Calculate the number of milliliters per hour.
$$1 \text{ min} : 1.2 \text{ ml} :: 60 \text{ min} : x \text{ ml}$$
$$x = 1.2 \times 60$$
$$x = 72 \text{ ml/hour}$$

32 Correct answer — **B**

D/A

$$\frac{\overset{7}{\cancel{35} \text{ gtt}}}{1 \text{ min}} \times \frac{1 \text{ ml}}{\underset{3}{\cancel{15} \text{ gtt}}} = \frac{7 \text{ ml}}{3 \text{ min}} = 2.3 \text{ ml/minute}$$

R/P

$$15 \text{ gtt} : 1 \text{ ml} :: 35 \text{ gtt} : x \text{ ml}$$
$$15x = 35$$
$$x = \frac{35}{15}$$
$$x = 2.3 \text{ ml/minute}$$

33 Correct answer — **B**

D/A

$$\frac{25 \text{ \cancel{mg}}}{1 \text{ hr}} \times \frac{\overset{1}{\cancel{250} \text{ ml}}}{\underset{2}{\cancel{500} \text{ \cancel{mg}}}} = \frac{25 \text{ ml}}{2 \text{ hr}} = 12.5 \text{ ml/hour}$$

R/P

$$500 \text{ mg} : 250 \text{ ml} :: 25 \text{ mg} : x \text{ ml}$$
$$500x = 250 \times 25$$
$$x = \frac{6,250}{500}$$
$$x = 12.5 \text{ ml/hour}$$

34 Correct answer — **A**

D/A

$$\frac{\overset{1}{\cancel{600} \text{ \cancel{U}}}}{1 \text{ hr}} \times \frac{250 \text{ ml}}{\underset{20}{\cancel{12,000} \text{ \cancel{U}}}} = \frac{250 \text{ ml}}{20 \text{ hr}} = 12.5 \text{ ml/hour}$$

R/P

$$12{,}000 \text{ U} : 250 \text{ ml} :: 600 \text{ U} : x \text{ ml}$$
$$12{,}000x = 250 \times 600$$
$$x = \frac{150{,}000}{12{,}000}$$
$$x = 12.5 \text{ ml/hour}$$

35 Correct answer—C

Remember: 1 mg = 1,000 mcg

D/A

$$\frac{\overset{1}{\cancel{4} \text{ mcg}}}{1 \text{ m\cancel{in}}} \times \frac{5\cancel{0}0 \text{ ml}}{\underset{\cancel{4}}{2{,}0\cancel{0}0 \text{ mcg}}} \times \frac{60 \text{ m\cancel{in}}}{1 \text{ hr}} = 60 \text{ ml/hour}$$

R/P

$$2{,}000 \text{ mcg} : 500 \text{ ml} :: 4 \text{ mcg} : x \text{ ml}$$
$$2{,}000x = 500 \times 4$$
$$x = \frac{2{,}000}{2{,}000}$$
$$x = 1 \text{ ml/minute or } 60 \text{ ml/hour}$$

36 Correct answer—C

D/A

$$400 \text{ m\cancel{l}} \times \frac{\overset{2}{2\cancel{0} \text{ gtt}}}{1 \text{ m\cancel{l}}} \times \frac{1 \text{ m\cancel{in}}}{\underset{5}{5\cancel{0} \text{ gtt}}} \times \frac{1 \text{ hr}}{60 \text{ m\cancel{in}}} =$$

$$\frac{800 \text{ hr}}{300} = 2.66 \text{ hours or 2 hours, 40 minutes}$$

R/P

Step 1: Change milliliters to drops.
$$1 \text{ ml} : 20 \text{ gtt} :: 400 \text{ ml} : x \text{ gtt}$$
$$x = 20 \times 400$$
$$x = 8{,}000 \text{ gtt}$$

Step 2: Calculate required minutes.

$$50 \text{ gtt} : 1 \text{ min} :: 8{,}000 \text{ gtt} : x \text{ min}$$
$$50x = 8{,}000$$
$$x = \frac{8{,}000}{50}$$
$$x = 160 \text{ minutes}$$

Step 3: Change minutes to hours.

$$60 \text{ min} : 1 \text{ hr} :: 160 \text{ min} : x \text{ hr}$$
$$60x = 160$$
$$x = \frac{160}{60}$$
$$x = 2.66 \text{ hours or 2 hours, 40 minutes}$$

37 Correct answer — **D**

D/A

$$\overset{10}{\cancel{2\cancel{5}0}} \; \cancel{\text{ml}} \times \frac{\overset{1}{\cancel{10} \text{ gtt}}}{1 \; \cancel{\text{ml}}} \times \frac{1 \; \cancel{\text{min}}}{\underset{1}{\cancel{25} \text{ gtt}}} \times \frac{1 \text{ hr}}{\underset{6}{\cancel{60} \; \cancel{\text{min}}}} =$$

$$\frac{10 \text{ hr}}{6} = 1.6 \text{ hours or 1 hour, 40 minutes}$$

The I.V. infusion will end at 9:40 a.m.

R/P

Step 1: Change milliliters to drops.

$$1 \text{ ml} : 10 \text{ gtt} :: 250 \text{ ml} : x \text{ gtt}$$
$$x = 10 \times 250$$
$$x = 2{,}500 \text{ gtt}$$

Step 2: Calculate required minutes.

$$25 \text{ gtt} : 1 \text{ min} :: 2{,}500 \text{ gtt} : x \text{ min}$$
$$25x = 2{,}500$$
$$x = \frac{2{,}500}{250}$$
$$x = 100 \text{ minutes or 1 hour, 40 minutes}$$

The I.V. infusion will end at 9:40 a.m.

38 Correct answer — **A**

D/A

$$\overset{2}{\cancel{3\cancel{0}0}} \; \cancel{\text{ml}} \times \frac{\overset{1}{\cancel{60} \text{ mcgtt}}}{1 \; \cancel{\text{ml}}} \times \frac{1 \; \cancel{\text{min}}}{\underset{1}{\cancel{150} \text{ mcgtt}}} \times \frac{1 \text{ hr}}{\underset{1}{\cancel{60} \; \cancel{\text{min}}}} = 2 \text{ hours}$$

The infusion will end at 4 p.m.

R/P

Step 1: Change milliliters to microdrops.

$$1 \text{ ml} : 60 \text{ mcgtt} :: 300 \text{ ml} : x \text{ mcgtt}$$
$$x = 60 \times 300$$
$$x = 18{,}000 \text{ mcgtt}$$

Step 2: Calculate required minutes.

$$150 \text{ mcgtt} : 1 \text{ min} :: 18{,}000 \text{ mcgtt} : x \text{ min}$$
$$150x = 18{,}000$$
$$x = \frac{18{,}000}{150}$$
$$x = 120 \text{ minutes or 2 hours}$$

The infusion will end at 4 p.m.

---

39 Correct answer — **C**

D/A

$$\overset{50}{\cancel{500}} \cancel{\text{ml}} \times \frac{\overset{1}{\cancel{15}} \cancel{\text{gtt}}}{1 \cancel{\text{ml}}} \times \frac{1 \cancel{\text{min}}}{\underset{1}{\cancel{10}} \cancel{\text{gtt}}} \times \frac{1 \text{ hr}}{\underset{4}{\cancel{60}} \cancel{\text{min}}} = \frac{50 \text{ hr}}{4} = 12\tfrac{1}{2} \text{ hours}$$

R/P

Step 1: Change milliliters to drops.

$$1 \text{ ml} : 15 \text{ gtt} :: 500 \text{ ml} : x \text{ gtt}$$
$$x = 15 \times 500$$
$$x = 7{,}500 \text{ gtt}$$

Step 2: Calculate required minutes.

$$10 \text{ gtt} : 1 \text{ min} :: 7{,}500 \text{ gtt} : x \text{ min}$$
$$10x = 7{,}500$$
$$x = \frac{7{,}500}{10}$$
$$x = 750 \text{ minutes}$$

Step 3: Change minutes to hours.

$$60 \text{ min} : 1 \text{ hr} :: 750 \text{ min} : x \text{ hr}$$
$$60x = 750$$
$$x = \frac{750}{60}$$
$$x = 12\tfrac{1}{2} \text{ hours}$$

40 Correct answer — **A**

D/A

$$75 \text{ ml} \times \frac{\overset{1}{\cancel{60} \text{ mcgtt}}}{1 \text{ ml}} \times \frac{1 \text{ min}}{30 \text{ mcgtt}} \times \frac{1 \text{ hr}}{\underset{1}{\cancel{60} \text{ min}}} = \frac{75 \text{ hr}}{30} = 2\frac{1}{2} \text{ hours}$$

R/P

Step 1: Change milliliters to microdrops.
$$1 \text{ ml} : 60 \text{ mcgtt} :: 75 \text{ ml} : x \text{ mcgtt}$$
$$x = 60 \times 75$$
$$x = 4{,}500 \text{ mcgtt}$$

Step 2: Calculate required minutes.
$$30 \text{ mcgtt} : 1 \text{ min} :: 4{,}500 \text{ mcgtt} : x \text{ min}$$
$$30x = 4{,}500$$
$$x = \frac{4{,}500}{30}$$
$$x = 150 \text{ minutes}$$

Step 3: Change minutes to hours.
$$60 \text{ min} : 1 \text{ hr} :: 150 \text{ min} : x \text{ hr}$$
$$60x = 150$$
$$x = \frac{150}{60}$$
$$x = 2\frac{1}{2} \text{ hours}$$

41 Correct answer — **D**

D/A

$$\overset{100}{\underset{}{1{,}000}} \text{ ml} \times \frac{\overset{1}{\cancel{60} \text{ mcgtt}}}{1 \text{ ml}} \times \frac{1 \text{ min}}{\underset{15}{150} \text{ mcgtt}} \times \frac{1 \text{ hr}}{\underset{1}{\cancel{60} \text{ min}}} =$$

$$\frac{100 \text{ hr}}{15} = 6.6 \text{ hours or 6 hours, 40 minutes}$$

R/P

Step 1: Change milliliters to microdrops.
$$1 \text{ ml} : 60 \text{ mcgtt} :: 1{,}000 \text{ ml} : x \text{ mcgtt}$$
$$x = 60 \times 1{,}000$$
$$x = 60{,}000 \text{ mcgtt}$$

Step 2: Calculate required minutes.

$$150 \text{ mcgtt} : 1 \text{ min} :: 60 \text{ mcgtt} : x \text{ min}$$
$$150x = 60,000$$
$$x = \frac{60,000}{150}$$
$$x = 400 \text{ minutes}$$

Step 3: Change minutes to hours.

$$60 \text{ min} : 1 \text{ hr} :: 400 \text{ min} : x \text{ hr}$$
$$60x = 400$$
$$x = \frac{400}{60}$$
$$x = 6.6 \text{ hours or 6 hours, 40 minutes}$$

42 Correct answer — **B**

Remember: 1 g = 1,000 mg

D/A

$$\frac{2 \ \cancel{\text{mg}}}{1 \text{ min}} \times \frac{\overset{1}{\cancel{500}} \ \cancel{\text{ml}}}{\underset{2}{\cancel{1,000}} \ \cancel{\text{mg}}} \times \frac{15 \text{ gtt}}{1 \ \cancel{\text{ml}}} = \frac{30 \text{ gtt}}{2 \text{ min}} = 15 \text{ gtt/minute}$$

R/P

Step 1: Change milliliters to drops.

$$1 \text{ ml} : 15 \text{ gtt} :: 500 \text{ ml} : x \text{ gtt}$$
$$x = 15 \times 500$$
$$x = 7,500 \text{ gtt}$$

Step 2: Calculate required minutes.

$$2 \text{ mg} : 1 \text{ min} :: 1,000 \text{ mg} : x \text{ min}$$
$$2x = 1,000$$
$$x = \frac{1,000}{2}$$
$$x = 500 \text{ minutes}$$

Step 3: Calculate the flow rate.

$$500 \text{ min} : 7,500 \text{ gtt} :: 1 \text{ min} : x \text{ gtt}$$
$$500x = 7,500$$
$$x = \frac{7,500}{500}$$
$$x = 15 \text{ gtt/minute}$$

43 Correct answer — **D**

D/A

$$\frac{0.3 \text{ mg}}{1 \text{ min}} \times \frac{\overset{5}{500} \text{ ml}}{\underset{1}{100} \text{ mg}} \times \frac{60 \text{ mcgtt}}{1 \text{ ml}} = 90 \text{ mcgtt/minute}$$

R/P

Step 1: Change milliliters to microdrops.
$$1 \text{ ml} : 60 \text{ mcgtt} :: 500 \text{ ml} : x \text{ mcgtt}$$
$$x = 60 \times 500$$
$$x = 30,000 \text{ mcgtt}$$

Step 2: Calculate required minutes.
$$0.3 \text{ mg} : 1 \text{ min} :: 100 \text{ mg} : x \text{ min}$$
$$0.3x = 100$$
$$x = \frac{100}{0.3}$$
$$x = 333.3 \text{ minutes}$$

Step 3: Calculate the flow rate.
$$333.3 \text{ min} : 30,000 \text{ mcgtt} :: 1 \text{ min} : x \text{ mcgtt}$$
$$333.3x = 30,000$$
$$x = \frac{30,000}{333.3}$$
$$x = 90 \text{ mcgtt/minute}$$

44 Correct answer — **A**
Remember: 1,000 mU = 1 U

D/A

$$\frac{600 \text{ mU}}{1 \text{ hr}} \times \frac{\overset{1}{1,000} \text{ ml}}{\underset{10}{10,000} \text{ mU}} \times \frac{\overset{1}{60} \text{ mcgtt}}{1 \text{ ml}} \times \frac{1 \text{ hr}}{\underset{1}{60} \text{ min}} = 60 \text{ mcgtt/minute}$$

R/P

Step 1: Change milliliters to microdrops.
$$1 \text{ ml} : 60 \text{ mcgtt} :: 1,000 \text{ ml} : x \text{ mcgtt}$$
$$x = 60 \times 1,000$$
$$x = 60,000 \text{ mcgtt}$$

Step 2: Calculate required minutes.

$$600 \text{ mU} : 60 \text{ min} :: 10,000 \text{ mU} : x \text{ min}$$
$$600x = 60 \times 10,000$$
$$x = \frac{60,000}{600}$$
$$x = 1,000 \text{ minutes}$$

Step 3: Calculate the flow rate.

$$1,000 \text{ min} : 60,000 \text{ mcgtt} :: 1 \text{ min} : x \text{ mcgtt}$$
$$1,000x = 60,000$$
$$x = \frac{60,000}{1,000}$$
$$x = 60 \text{ mcgtt/minute}$$

45 Correct answer—**B**

Remember: 1 gr = 60 mg

D/A

$$\frac{1 \ \cancel{mg}}{\cancel{10} \ \text{min}} \times \frac{\overset{100}{\cancel{1,000}} \ \cancel{ml}}{\underset{6}{\cancel{60}} \ \cancel{mg}} \times \frac{\overset{2}{\cancel{20}} \ \text{gtt}}{1 \ \cancel{ml}} = \frac{200 \text{ gtt}}{6 \text{ min}} = 33.3 \text{ or } 33 \text{ gtt/minute}$$

R/P

Step 1: Change milliliters to drops.

$$1 \text{ ml} : 20 \text{ gtt} :: 1,000 \text{ ml} : x \text{ gtt}$$
$$x = 20 \times 1,000$$
$$x = 20,000 \text{ gtt}$$

Step 2: Calculate required minutes.

$$1 \text{ mg} : 10 \text{ min} :: 60 \text{ mg} : x \text{ min}$$
$$x = 10 \times 60$$
$$x = 600 \text{ minutes}$$

Step 3: Calculate the flow rate.

$$600 \text{ min} : 20,000 \text{ gtt} :: 1 \text{ min} : x \text{ gtt}$$
$$600x = 20,000$$
$$x = \frac{20,000}{600}$$
$$x = 33.3 \text{ or } 33 \text{ gtt/minute}$$

46 Correct answer—**A**

D/A

$$\frac{0.35 \ \cancel{mg}}{1 \ \text{min}} \times \frac{\overset{10}{\cancel{500}} \ \cancel{ml}}{\underset{3}{\cancel{150}} \ \cancel{mg}} \times \frac{20 \text{ gtt}}{1 \ \cancel{ml}} = \frac{70 \text{ gtt}}{3 \text{ min}} = 23.3 \text{ or } 23 \text{ gtt/minute}$$

R/P

Step 1: Change milliliters to drops.

$$1 \text{ ml} : 20 \text{ gtt} :: 500 \text{ ml} : x \text{ gtt}$$
$$x = 20 \times 500$$
$$x = 10,000 \text{ gtt}$$

Step 2: Calculate required minutes.

$$0.35 \text{ mg} : 1 \text{ min} :: 150 \text{ mg} : x \text{ min}$$
$$0.35x = 150$$
$$x = \frac{150}{0.35}$$
$$x = 428.6 \text{ minutes}$$

Step 3: Calculate flow rate.

$$428.6 \text{ min} : 10,000 \text{ gtt} :: 1 \text{ min} : x \text{ gtt}$$
$$428.6x = 10,000$$
$$x = \frac{10,000}{428.6}$$
$$x = 23.3 \text{ or } 23 \text{ gtt/minute}$$

---

47 Correct answer — **A**

D/A

$$\frac{\overset{1}{\cancel{500,000}} \, \cancel{U}}{\underset{4}{\cancel{60} \text{ min}}} \times \frac{1,000 \, \cancel{ml}}{\underset{10}{\cancel{5,000,000}} \, \cancel{U}} \times \frac{\overset{1}{\cancel{15}} \text{ gtt}}{1 \, \cancel{ml}} = \frac{1,000 \text{ gtt}}{40 \text{ min}} = 25 \text{ gtt/minute}$$

R/P

Step 1: Change milliliters to drops.

$$1 \text{ ml} : 15 \text{ gtt} :: 1,000 \text{ ml} : x \text{ gtt}$$
$$x = 15 \times 1,000$$
$$x = 15,000 \text{ gtt}$$

Step 2: Calculate required minutes.

$$500,000 \text{ U} : 60 \text{ min} :: 5,000,000 \text{ U} : x \text{ min}$$
$$500,000x = 60 \times 5,000,000$$
$$x = \frac{300,000,000}{500,000}$$
$$x = 600 \text{ minutes}$$

Step 3: Calculate the flow rate.

$$600 \text{ min} : 15,000 \text{ gtt} :: 1 \text{ min} : x \text{ gtt}$$
$$600x = 15,000$$
$$x = \frac{15,000}{600}$$
$$x = 25 \text{ gtt/minute}$$

48 Correct answer—**C**

D/A

$$\frac{0.05 \; \cancel{mg}}{1 \; min} \times \frac{500 \; \cancel{ml}}{\underset{1}{\cancel{10} \; \cancel{mg}}} \times \frac{\overset{1}{\cancel{10} \; gtt}}{1 \; \cancel{ml}} = 25 \; gtt/minute$$

R/P

Step 1: Change milliliters to drops.

$$1 \; ml : 10 \; gtt :: 500 \; ml : x \; gtt$$
$$x = 10 \times 500$$
$$x = 5,000 \; gtt$$

Step 2: Calculate required minutes.

$$0.05 \; mg : 1 \; min :: 10 \; mg : x \; min$$
$$0.05x = 10$$
$$x = \frac{10}{0.05}$$
$$x = 200 \; minutes$$

Step 3: Calculate the flow rate.

$$200 \; min : 5,000 \; gtt :: 1 \; min : x \; gtt$$
$$200x = 5,000$$
$$x = \frac{5,000}{200}$$
$$x = 25 \; gtt/minute$$

49 Correct answer—**C**

D/A

$$\frac{\overset{1}{\cancel{5} \; \cancel{mEq}}}{\underset{1}{\cancel{60} \; min}} \times \frac{500 \; \cancel{ml}}{\underset{8}{\cancel{40} \; \cancel{mEq}}} \times \frac{\overset{1}{\cancel{60} \; mcgtt}}{1 \; \cancel{ml}} =$$

$$\frac{500 \; mcgtt}{8 \; min} = 62.5 \; or \; 63 \; mcgtt/minute$$

R/P

Step 1: Change milliliters to microdrops.

$$1 \text{ ml} : 60 \text{ mcgtt} :: 500 \text{ ml} : x \text{ mcgtt}$$
$$x = 60 \times 500$$
$$x = 30,000 \text{ mcgtt}$$

Step 2: Calculate required minutes.

$$5 \text{ mEq} : 60 \text{ min} :: 40 \text{ mEq} : x \text{ min}$$
$$5x = 60 \times 40$$
$$x = \frac{2,400}{5}$$
$$x = 480 \text{ minutes}$$

Step 3: Calculate flow rate.

$$480 \text{ min} : 30,000 \text{ mcgtt} :: 1 \text{ min} : x \text{ mcgtt}$$
$$480x = 30,000$$
$$x = \frac{30,000}{480}$$
$$x = 62.5 \text{ or } 63 \text{ mcgtt/minute}$$

---

50 Correct answer — **B**

D/A

$$\frac{2.5 \text{ mg}}{60 \text{ min}} \times \frac{\overset{50}{\cancel{500}} \text{ ml}}{\underset{3}{\cancel{30}} \text{ mg}} \times \frac{\cancel{20} \text{ gtt}}{1 \text{ ml}} = \frac{250 \text{ gtt}}{18 \text{ min}} = 13.8 \text{ or } 14 \text{ gtt/minute}$$

R/P

Step 1: Change milliliters to drops.

$$1 \text{ ml} : 20 \text{ gtt} :: 500 \text{ ml} : x \text{ gtt}$$
$$x = 20 \times 500$$
$$x = 10,000 \text{ gtt}$$

Step 2: Calculate required minutes.

$$2.5 \text{ mg} : 60 \text{ min} :: 30 \text{ mg} : x \text{ min}$$
$$2.5x = 60 \times 30$$
$$x = \frac{1,800}{2.5}$$
$$x = 720 \text{ minutes}$$

Step 3: Calculate the flow rate.

$$720 \text{ min} : 10,000 \text{ gtt} :: 1 \text{ min} : x \text{ gtt}$$
$$720x = 10,000$$
$$x = \frac{10,000}{720}$$
$$x = 13.8 \text{ or } 14 \text{ gtt/minute}$$

51 Correct answer — **B**

D/A

$$\frac{2.5 \text{ mg}}{1 \text{ min}} \times \frac{\overset{2}{100 \text{ ml}}}{\underset{1}{50 \text{ mg}}} \times \frac{10 \text{ gtt}}{1 \text{ ml}} = 50 \text{ gtt/minute}$$

R/P

Step 1: Change milliliters to drops.

$$1 \text{ ml} : 10 \text{ gtt} :: 100 \text{ ml} : x \text{ gtt}$$
$$x = 10 \times 100$$
$$x = 1{,}000 \text{ gtt}$$

Step 2: Calculate required minutes.

$$2.5 \text{ mg} : 1 \text{ min} :: 50 \text{ mg} : x \text{ min}$$
$$2.5x = 50$$
$$x = \frac{50}{2.5}$$
$$x = 20 \text{ minutes}$$

Step 3: Calculate the flow rate.

$$20 \text{ min} : 1{,}000 \text{ gtt} :: 1 \text{ min} : x \text{ gtt}$$
$$20x = 1{,}000$$
$$x = \frac{1{,}000}{20}$$
$$x = 50 \text{ gtt/minute}$$

52 Correct answer — **D**

D/A

$$\frac{5 \text{ mg}}{1 \text{ min}} \times \frac{\overset{1}{250 \text{ ml}}}{\underset{2}{500 \text{ mg}}} \times \frac{20 \text{ gtt}}{1 \text{ ml}} = \frac{100 \text{ gtt}}{2 \text{ min}} = 50 \text{ gtt/minute}$$

R/P

Step 1: Change milliliters to drops.

$$1 \text{ ml} : 20 \text{ gtt} :: 250 \text{ ml} : x \text{ gtt}$$
$$x = 20 \times 250$$
$$x = 5{,}000 \text{ gtt}$$

Step 2: Calculate required minutes.

$$5 \text{ mg} : 1 \text{ min} :: 500 \text{ mg} : x \text{ min}$$
$$5x = 500$$
$$x = \frac{500}{5}$$
$$x = 100 \text{ minutes}$$

Step 3: Calculate the flow rate.

$$100 \text{ min} : 5,000 \text{ gtt} :: 1 \text{ min} : x \text{ gtt}$$
$$100x = 5,000$$
$$x = \frac{5,000}{100}$$
$$x = 50 \text{ gtt/minute}$$

53 Correct answer — A

D/A

$$\overset{1}{\underset{3}{\frac{50 \text{ mg}}{90 \text{ sec}}}} \times \overset{}{\underset{2}{\frac{10 \text{ ml}}{100 \text{ mg}}}} \times \frac{20 \text{ gtt}}{1 \text{ ml}} \times \overset{2}{\frac{60 \text{ sec}}{1 \text{ min}}} =$$

$$\frac{400 \text{ gtt}}{6 \text{ min}} = 66.6 \text{ or } 67 \text{ gtt/minute}$$

R/P

Step 1: Change milliliters to drops.

$$1 \text{ ml} : 20 \text{ gtt} :: 10 \text{ ml} : x \text{ gtt}$$
$$x = 20 \times 10$$
$$x = 200 \text{ gtt}$$

Step 2: Calculate required minutes.

$$50 \text{ mg} : 90 \text{ sec} :: 100 \text{ mg} : x \text{ sec}$$
$$50x = 90 \times 100$$
$$x = \frac{9,000}{50}$$
$$x = 180 \text{ seconds or } 3 \text{ minutes}$$

Step 3: Calculate the flow rate.

$$3 \text{ min} : 200 \text{ gtt} :: 1 \text{ min} : x \text{ gtt}$$
$$3x = 200$$
$$x = \frac{200}{3}$$
$$x = 66.6 \text{ or } 67 \text{ gtt/minute}$$

54 Correct answer — D

D/A

$$\overset{1}{\underset{1}{\frac{60 \text{ mg}}{60 \text{ min}}}} \times \overset{2}{\underset{3}{\frac{1,000 \text{ ml}}{1,500 \text{ mg}}}} \times \frac{20 \text{ gtt}}{1 \text{ ml}} = \frac{40 \text{ gtt}}{3 \text{ min}} = 13.3 \text{ or } 13 \text{ gtt/minute}$$

R/P

Step 1: Change milliliters to drops.
$$1 \text{ ml} : 20 \text{ gtt} :: 1{,}000 \text{ ml} : x \text{ gtt}$$
$$x = 20 \times 1{,}000$$
$$x = 20{,}000 \text{ gtt}$$

Step 2: Calculate required minutes.
$$60 \text{ mg} : 60 \text{ min} :: 1{,}500 \text{ mg} : x \text{ min}$$
$$x = 1{,}500 \text{ minutes}$$

Step 3: Calculate the flow rate.
$$1{,}500 \text{ min} : 20{,}000 \text{ gtt} :: 1 \text{ min} : x \text{ gtt}$$
$$1{,}500x = 20{,}000$$
$$x = \frac{20{,}000}{1{,}500}$$
$$x = 13.3 \text{ or } 13 \text{ gtt/minute}$$

55 Correct answer — **B**

D/A

$$\frac{4 \text{ mg}}{60 \text{ min}} \times \frac{100 \text{ ml}}{45 \text{ mg}} \times \frac{\overset{1}{60} \text{ mcgtt}}{1 \text{ ml}} =$$

$$\frac{400 \text{ mcgtt}}{45 \text{ min}} = 8.8 \text{ or } 9 \text{ mcgtt/minute}$$

R/P

Step 1: Change milliliters to microdrops.
$$1 \text{ ml} : 60 \text{ mcgtt} :: 100 \text{ ml} : x \text{ mcgtt}$$
$$x = 60 \times 100$$
$$x = 6{,}000 \text{ mcgtt}$$

Step 2: Calculate required minutes.
$$4 \text{ mg} : 60 \text{ min} :: 45 \text{ mg} : x \text{ min}$$
$$4x = 60 \times 45$$
$$x = \frac{2{,}700}{4}$$
$$x = 675 \text{ minutes}$$

Step 3: Calculate the flow rate.
$$675 \text{ min} : 600 \text{ mcgtt} :: 1 \text{ min} : x \text{ mcgtt}$$
$$675x = 6{,}000$$
$$x = \frac{6{,}000}{675}$$
$$x = 8.8 \text{ or } 9 \text{ mcgtt/minute}$$

56 Correct answer — **D**

D/A

$$\frac{2 \text{ mg}}{1 \text{ min}} \times \frac{\overset{2}{\cancel{500}} \text{ ml}}{\underset{1}{\cancel{250}} \text{ mg}} \times \frac{15 \text{ gtt}}{1 \text{ ml}} = 60 \text{ gtt/minute}$$

R/P

Step 1: Change milliliters to drops.

$$1 \text{ ml} : 15 \text{ gtt} :: 50 \text{ ml} : x \text{ gtt}$$
$$x = 15 \times 500$$
$$x = 7,500 \text{ gtt}$$

Step 2: Calculate required minutes.

$$2 \text{ mg} : 1 \text{ min} :: 250 \text{ mg} : x \text{ min}$$
$$2x = 250$$
$$x = \frac{250}{2}$$
$$x = 125 \text{ minutes}$$

Step 3: Calculate the flow rate.

$$125 \text{ min} : 7,500 \text{ gtt} :: 1 \text{ min} : x \text{ gtt}$$
$$125x = 7,500$$
$$x = \frac{7,500}{125}$$
$$x = 60 \text{ gtt/minute}$$

57 Correct answer — **B**

D/A

$$\frac{6 \text{ mg}}{1 \text{ min}} \times \frac{\overset{1}{\cancel{100}} \text{ ml}}{\underset{5}{\cancel{500}} \text{ mg}} \times \frac{10 \text{ gtt}}{1 \text{ ml}} = \frac{60 \text{ gtt}}{5 \text{ min}} = 12 \text{ gtt/minute}$$

R/P

Step 1: Change milliliters to drops.

$$1 \text{ ml} : 10 \text{ gtt} :: 100 \text{ ml} : x \text{ gtt}$$
$$x = 10 \times 100$$
$$x = 1,000 \text{ gtt}$$

Step 2: Calculate required minutes.

$$6 \text{ mg} : 1 \text{ min} :: 500 \text{ mg} : x \text{ min}$$
$$60x = 500$$
$$x = \frac{500}{6}$$
$$x = 83.3 \text{ minutes}$$

Step 3: Calculate the flow rate.

$$83.3 \text{ min} : 1{,}000 \text{ gtt} :: 1 \text{ min} : x \text{ gtt}$$
$$83.3x = 1{,}000$$
$$x = \frac{1{,}000}{83.3}$$
$$x = 12 \text{ gtt/minute}$$

58 Correct answer — **B**

Remember: 1 g = 1,000 mg

D/A

$$\frac{30 \text{ m\cancel{g}}}{1 \text{ min}} \times \frac{\overset{1}{\cancel{50}} \text{ m\cancel{l}}}{\underset{20}{\cancel{1{,}000}} \text{ m\cancel{g}}} \times \frac{60 \text{ mcgtt}}{1 \text{ m\cancel{l}}} = \frac{1{,}800 \text{ mcgtt}}{20 \text{ min}} = 90 \text{ mcgtt/minute}$$

R/P

Step 1: Change milliliters to microdrops.

$$1 \text{ ml} : 60 \text{ mcgtt} :: 50 \text{ ml} : x \text{ mcgtt}$$
$$x = 60 \times 50$$
$$x = 3{,}000 \text{ mcgtt}$$

Step 2: Calculate required minutes.

$$30 \text{ mg} : 1 \text{ min} :: 1{,}000 \text{ mg} : x \text{ min}$$
$$30x = 1{,}000$$
$$x = \frac{1{,}000}{30}$$
$$x = 33.3 \text{ minutes}$$

Step 3: Calculate the flow rate.

$$33.3 \text{ min} : 3{,}000 \text{ mcgtt} :: 1 \text{ min} : x \text{ mcgtt}$$
$$33.3x = 3{,}000$$
$$x = \frac{3{,}000}{33.3}$$
$$x = 90 \text{ mcgtt/minute}$$

59 Correct answer — **A**

D/A

$$\frac{3 \text{ m\cancel{g}}}{1 \text{ min}} \times \frac{\overset{1}{\cancel{500}} \text{ m\cancel{l}}}{\underset{4}{\cancel{2{,}000}} \text{ m\cancel{g}}} \times \frac{20 \text{ gtt}}{1 \text{ m\cancel{l}}} = \frac{60 \text{ gtt}}{4 \text{ min}} = 15 \text{ gtt/minute}$$

R/P

Step 1: Change milliliters to drops.

$$1 \text{ ml} : 20 \text{ gtt} :: 50 \text{ ml} : x \text{ gtt}$$
$$x = 20 \times 500$$
$$x = 10,000 \text{ gtt}$$

Step 2: Calculate required minutes.

$$3 \text{ mg} : 1 \text{ min} :: 2,000 \text{ mg} : x \text{ min}$$
$$3x = 2,000$$
$$x = \frac{2,000}{3}$$
$$x = 666.6 \text{ minutes}$$

Step 3: Calculate the flow rate.

$$666.6 \text{ min} : 10,000 \text{ gtt} :: 1 \text{ min} : x \text{ gtt}$$
$$666.6x = 10,000$$
$$x = \frac{10,000}{666.6}$$
$$x = 15 \text{ gtt/minute}$$

---

60 Correct answer — **C**

D/A

$$\frac{\overset{1}{\cancel{250} \text{ mg}}}{\underset{4}{\cancel{60} \text{ min}}} \times \frac{250 \text{ ml}}{\underset{4}{\cancel{1,000} \text{ mg}}} \times \frac{\overset{1}{\cancel{15} \text{ gtt}}}{1 \text{ ml}} = \frac{250 \text{ gtt}}{16 \text{ min}} = 15.6 \text{ or } 16 \text{ gtt/minute}$$

R/P

Step 1: Change milliliters to drops.

$$1 \text{ ml} : 15 \text{ gtt} :: 250 \text{ ml} : x \text{ gtt}$$
$$x = 15 \times 250$$
$$x = 3,750 \text{ gtt}$$

Step 2: Calculate required minutes.

$$250 \text{ mg} : 60 \text{ min} :: 1,000 \text{ mg} : x \text{ min}$$
$$250x = 60 \times 1,000$$
$$x = \frac{60,000}{250}$$
$$x = 240 \text{ minutes}$$

Step 3: Calculate the flow rate.

$$240 \text{ min} : 3,750 \text{ gtt} :: 1 \text{ min} : x \text{ gtt}$$
$$240x = 3,750$$
$$x = \frac{3,750}{240}$$
$$x = 15.6 \text{ or } 16 \text{ gtt/minute}$$

61 Correct answer — **D**

D/A

$$\frac{\overset{10}{\cancel{50}\ \cancel{ml}}}{\underset{1}{\cancel{5}\ min}} \times \frac{10\ gtt}{1\ \cancel{ml}} = 100\ gtt/minute$$

R/P

Step 1: Change milliliters to drops.

$$1\ ml : 10\ gtt :: 50\ ml : x\ gtt$$
$$x = 10 \times 50$$
$$x = 500\ gtt$$

Step 2: Calculate the flow rate.

$$5\ min : 500\ gtt :: 1\ min : x\ gtt$$
$$5x = 500$$
$$x = \frac{500}{5}$$
$$x = 100\ gtt/minute$$

62 Correct answer — **A**

D/A

$$\frac{1.25\ \cancel{mg}}{\underset{3}{\cancel{60}\ min}} \times \frac{\overset{100}{1,\cancel{000}\ \cancel{ml}}}{\underset{1}{\cancel{10}\ \cancel{mg}}} \times \frac{\overset{1}{\cancel{20}\ gtt}}{1\ \cancel{ml}} = \frac{125\ gtt}{3\ min} = 41.6\ or\ 42\ gtt/minute$$

R/P

Step 1: Change milliliters to drops.

$$1\ ml : 20\ gtt :: 1,000\ ml : x\ gtt$$
$$x = 20 \times 1,000$$
$$x = 20,000\ gtt$$

Step 2: Calculate required minutes.

$$1.25\ mg : 60\ min :: 10\ mg : x\ min$$
$$1.25x = 60 \times 10$$
$$x = \frac{600}{1.25}$$
$$x = 480\ minutes$$

Step 3: Calculate the flow rate.

$$480\ min : 20,000\ gtt :: 1\ min : x\ gtt$$
$$480x = 20,000$$
$$x = \frac{20,000}{480}$$
$$x = 41.6\ or\ 42\ gtt/minute$$

63 Correct answer — **D**

D/A

$$\frac{600 \text{ m\!/g}}{\underset{3}{6\!\!/0} \text{ min}} \times \frac{1 \text{ \!/g}}{\underset{5}{1,0\!\!/0\!\!/0 \text{ m\!/g}}} \times \frac{\overset{1}{2\!\!/0\!\!/0} \text{ m\!/l}}{1.2 \text{ \!/g}} \times \frac{\overset{1}{2\!\!/0} \text{ gtt}}{1 \text{ m\!/l}} =$$

$$\frac{600 \text{ gtt}}{18 \text{ min}} = 33.3 \text{ or } 33 \text{ gtt/minute}$$

R/P

Step 1: Change milliliters to drops.

$$1 \text{ ml} : 20 \text{ gtt} :: 200 \text{ ml} : x \text{ gtt}$$
$$x = 20 \times 200$$
$$x = 4,000 \text{ gtt}$$

Step 2: Change grams to milligrams.

$$1 \text{ g} : 1,000 \text{ mg} :: 1.2 \text{ g} : x \text{ mg}$$
$$x = 1,000 \times 1.2$$
$$x = 1,200 \text{ mg}$$

Step 3: Calculate required minutes.

$$600 \text{ mg} : 60 \text{ min} :: 1,200 \text{ mg} : x \text{ min}$$
$$600x = 60 \times 1,200$$
$$x = \frac{72,000}{600}$$
$$x = 120 \text{ minutes}$$

Step 4: Calculate the flow rate.

$$120 \text{ min} : 4,000 \text{ gtt} :: 1 \text{ min} : x \text{ gtt}$$
$$120x = 4,000$$
$$x = \frac{4,000}{120}$$
$$x = 33.3 \text{ or } 33 \text{ gtt/minute}$$

64 Correct answer — **D**

D/A

$$\frac{\underset{10}{1,0\!\!/0\!\!/0 \text{ m\!/l}}}{\overset{1}{10,0\!\!/0\!\!/0 \text{ \!/U}}} \times \frac{250 \text{ \!/U}}{\underset{1}{6\!\!/0} \text{ min}} \times \frac{\overset{1}{6\!\!/0} \text{ mcgtt}}{1 \text{ m\!/l}} = \frac{250 \text{ mcgtt}}{10 \text{ min}} = 25 \text{ mcgtt/minute}$$

R/P

Step 1: Change milliliters to drops.

$$1 \text{ ml} : 60 \text{ mcgtt} :: 1,000 \text{ ml} : x \text{ mcgtt}$$
$$x = 60 \times 1,000$$
$$x = 60,000 \text{ mcgtt}$$

Step 2: Calculate required minutes.

$$250 \text{ U} : 60 \text{ min} :: 10{,}000 \text{ U} : x \text{ min}$$
$$250x = 600{,}000$$
$$x = \frac{600{,}000}{250}$$
$$x = 2{,}400 \text{ minutes}$$

Step 3: Calculate the flow rate.

$$2{,}400 \text{ min} : 60{,}000 \text{ mcgtt} :: 1 \text{ min} : x \text{ mcgtt}$$
$$2{,}400x = 60{,}000$$
$$x = \frac{60{,}000}{2{,}400}$$
$$x = 25 \text{ mcgtt/minute}$$

65 Correct answer — B

D/A

$$\frac{\overset{1}{\cancel{400 \cancel{U}}}}{\underset{1}{\cancel{60} \text{ min}}} \times \frac{\overset{1}{1{,}\cancel{000} \cancel{ml}}}{\underset{10}{10{,}\cancel{000} \cancel{U}}} \times \frac{\overset{1}{\cancel{60} \text{ mcgtt}}}{1 \cancel{ml}} =$$

$$\frac{400 \text{ mcgtt}}{10 \text{ min}} = 40 \text{ mcgtt/minute}$$

R/P

Step 1: Change milliliters to microdrops.

$$1 \text{ ml} : 60 \text{ mcgtt} :: 1{,}000 \text{ ml} : x \text{ mcgtt}$$
$$x = 60 \times 1{,}000$$
$$x = 60{,}000 \text{ mcgtt}$$

Step 2: Calculate required minutes.

$$400 \text{ U} : 60 \text{ min} :: 10{,}000 \text{ U} : x \text{ min}$$
$$400x = 60 \times 10{,}000$$
$$x = \frac{600{,}000}{400}$$
$$x = 1{,}500 \text{ minutes}$$

Step 3: Calculate the flow rate.

$$1{,}500 \text{ min} : 60{,}000 \text{ mcgtt} :: 1 \text{ min} : x \text{ mcgtt}$$
$$1{,}500x = 60{,}000$$
$$x = \frac{60{,}000}{1{,}500}$$
$$x = 40 \text{ mcgtt/minute}$$

66 Correct answer—**C**

D/A

$$\frac{0.35 \ \cancel{\text{mg}}}{1 \ \text{min}} \times \frac{\overset{5}{\cancel{1,000 \ \text{ml}}}}{\underset{1}{\cancel{200 \ \text{mg}}}} \times \frac{15 \ \text{gtt}}{1 \ \cancel{\text{ml}}} = 26.2 \ \text{or 26 gtt/minute}$$

R/P

Step 1: Change milliliters to drops.

1 ml : 15 gtt :: 1,000 ml : x gtt

$$x = 15 \times 1,000$$
$$x = 15,000 \ \text{gtt}$$

Step 2: Calculate required minutes.

0.35 mg : 1 min :: 200 mg : x min

$$0.35x = 200$$
$$x = \frac{200}{0.35}$$
$$x = 571 \ \text{minutes}$$

Step 3: Calculate the flow rate.

571 min : 15,000 gtt :: 1 min : x gtt

$$571x = 15,000$$
$$x = \frac{15,000}{571}$$
$$x = 26.2 \ \text{or 26 gtt/minute}$$

67 Correct answer—**B**

Remember: 1 mg = 1,000 mcg

D/A

$$\frac{1 \ \cancel{\text{mcg}}}{1 \ \text{min}} \times \frac{\overset{1}{\cancel{250 \ \text{ml}}}}{\underset{4}{\cancel{1,000 \ \text{mcg}}}} \times \frac{60 \ \text{mcgtt}}{1 \ \cancel{\text{ml}}} = \frac{60 \ \text{mcgtt}}{4 \ \text{min}} = 15 \ \text{mcgtt/minute}$$

R/P

Step 1: Change milliliters to microdrops.

1 ml : 60 mcgtt :: 250 ml : x mcgtt

$$x = 60 \times 250$$
$$x = 15,000 \ \text{mcgtt}$$

Step 2: Calculate required minutes.

1 mcg : 1 min :: 1,000 mcg : x min

$$x = 1,000 \ \text{minutes}$$

Step 3: Calculate the flow rate.

$$1{,}000 \text{ min} : 15{,}000 \text{ mcgtt} :: 1 \text{ min} : x \text{ mcgtt}$$
$$1{,}000x = 15{,}000$$
$$x = \frac{15{,}000}{1{,}000}$$
$$x = 15 \text{ mcgtt/minute}$$

68 Correct answer — **A**

Remember: 1 g = 1,000 mg

D/A

$$\frac{4 \text{ mg}}{1 \text{ min}} \times \frac{\overset{1}{2{,}50} \text{ ml}}{\underset{4}{1{,}000} \text{ mg}} \times \frac{20 \text{ gtt}}{1 \text{ ml}} = \frac{80 \text{ gtt}}{4 \text{ min}} = 20 \text{ gtt/minute}$$

R/P

Step 1: Change milliliters to drops.

$$1 \text{ ml} : 20 \text{ gtt} :: 250 \text{ ml} : x \text{ gtt}$$
$$x = 20 \times 250$$
$$x = 5{,}000 \text{ gtt}$$

Step 2: Calculate required minutes.

$$4 \text{ mg} : 1 \text{ min} :: 1{,}000 \text{ mg} : x \text{ min}$$
$$4x = 1{,}000$$
$$x = \frac{1{,}000}{4}$$
$$x = 250 \text{ minutes}$$

Step 3: Calculate the flow rate.

$$250 \text{ min} : 5{,}000 \text{ gtt} :: 1 \text{ min} : x \text{ gtt}$$
$$250x = 5{,}000$$
$$x = \frac{5{,}000}{250}$$
$$x = 20 \text{ gtt/minute}$$

69 Correct answer — **C**

D/A

$$\frac{0.3 \text{ mg}}{1 \text{ min}} \times \frac{\overset{50}{5{,}00} \text{ ml}}{\underset{12}{1{,}20} \text{ mg}} \times \frac{10 \text{ gtt}}{1 \text{ ml}} = \frac{150 \text{ gtt}}{12 \text{ min}} = 12.5 \text{ or } 13 \text{ gtt/minute}$$

R/P

Step 1: Change milliliters to drops.

$$1 \text{ ml} : 10 \text{ gtt} :: 500 \text{ ml} : x \text{ gtt}$$
$$x = 10 \times 500$$
$$x = 5{,}000 \text{ gtt}$$

Step 2: Calculate required minutes.

$$0.3 \text{ mg} : 1 \text{ min} :: 120 \text{ mg} : x \text{ min}$$
$$0.3x = 120$$
$$x = \frac{120}{0.3}$$
$$x = 400 \text{ minutes}$$

Step 3: Calculate the flow rate.

$$400 \text{ min} : 5{,}000 \text{ gtt} :: 1 \text{ min} : x \text{ gtt}$$
$$400x = 5{,}000$$
$$x = \frac{5{,}000}{400}$$
$$x = 12.5 \text{ or } 13 \text{ gtt/minute}$$

70 Correct answer — **D**

D/A

$$\frac{0.12 \cancel{g}}{\underset{3}{\cancel{60}} \text{ min}} \times \frac{500 \cancel{ml}}{1 \cancel{g}} \times \frac{\overset{1}{\cancel{20}} \text{ gtt}}{1 \cancel{ml}} = \frac{60 \text{ gtt}}{3 \text{ min}} = 20 \text{ gtt/minute}$$

R/P

Step 1: Change milliliters to drops.

$$1 \text{ ml} : 20 \text{ gtt} :: 500 \text{ ml} : x \text{ gtt}$$
$$x = 20 \times 500$$
$$x = 10{,}000 \text{ gtt}$$

Step 2: Calculate required minutes.

$$0.12 \text{ g} : 60 \text{ min} :: 1 \text{ g} : x \text{ min}$$
$$0.12x = 60$$
$$x = \frac{60}{0.12}$$
$$x = 500 \text{ minutes}$$

Step 3: Calculate the flow rate.

$$500 \text{ min} : 10{,}000 \text{ gtt} :: 1 \text{ min} : x \text{ gtt}$$
$$500x = 10{,}000$$
$$x = \frac{10{,}000}{500}$$
$$x = 20 \text{ gtt/minute}$$

71 Correct answer – **A**

D/A

$$\frac{0.5 \overset{}{\underset{4}{\cancel{g}}}}{\underset{1}{\cancel{60}} \text{ min}} \times \frac{\overset{250}{\cancel{500}} \text{ ml}}{\underset{1}{\cancel{2}} \cancel{g}} \times \frac{\overset{1}{\cancel{15}} \text{ gtt}}{1 \cancel{\text{ml}}} = \frac{125 \text{ gtt}}{4 \text{ min}} = 31.2 \text{ or } 31 \text{ gtt/minute}$$

R/P

Step 1: Change milliliters to drops.

$$1 \text{ ml} : 15 \text{ gtt} :: 500 \text{ ml} : x \text{ gtt}$$
$$x = 15 \times 500$$
$$x = 7,500 \text{ gtt}$$

Step 2: Calculate required minutes.

$$0.5 \text{ g} : 60 \text{ min} :: 2 \text{ g} : x \text{ min}$$
$$0.5x = 60 \times 2$$
$$x = \frac{120}{0.5}$$
$$x = 240 \text{ minutes}$$

Step 3: Calculate the flow rate.

$$240 \text{ min} : 7,500 \text{ gtt} :: 1 \text{ min} : x \text{ gtt}$$
$$240x = 7,500$$
$$x = \frac{7,500}{240}$$
$$x = 31.2 \text{ or } 31 \text{ gtt/minute}$$

72 Correct answer – **C**

D/A

$$\frac{1 \cancel{g}}{\underset{1}{\cancel{60}} \text{ min}} \times \frac{\overset{50}{\cancel{100}} \text{ ml}}{\underset{1}{\cancel{2}} \cancel{g}} \times \frac{\overset{1}{\cancel{60}} \text{ mcgtt}}{1 \cancel{\text{ml}}} = 50 \text{ mcgtt/minute}$$

R/P

Step 1: Change milliliters to microdrops.

$$1 \text{ ml} : 60 \text{ mcgtt} :: 100 \text{ ml} : x \text{ mcgtt}$$
$$x = 60 \times 100$$
$$x = 6,000 \text{ mcgtt}$$

Step 2: Calculate required minutes.

$$1 \text{ g} : 60 \text{ min} :: 2 \text{ g} : x \text{ min}$$
$$x = 60 \times 2$$
$$x = 120 \text{ minutes}$$

Step 3: Calculate the flow rate.

$$120 \text{ min} : 6{,}000 \text{ mcgtt} :: 1 \text{ min} : x \text{ mcgtt}$$
$$120x = 6{,}000$$
$$x = \frac{6{,}000}{120}$$
$$x = 50 \text{ mcgtt/minute}$$

73 Correct answer — **D**

D/A

$$\frac{500 \, \cancel{U}}{\underset{3}{\cancel{60}} \text{ min}} \times \frac{\overset{1}{\cancel{1{,}000}} \, \cancel{ml}}{\underset{10}{\cancel{10{,}000}} \, \cancel{U}} \times \frac{\overset{1}{\cancel{20}} \text{ gtt}}{1 \, \cancel{ml}} = \frac{50 \text{ gtt}}{3 \text{ min}} = 16.6 \text{ or } 17 \text{ gtt/minute}$$

R/P

Step 1: Change milliliters to drops.

$$1 \text{ ml} : 20 \text{ gtt} :: 1{,}000 \text{ ml} : x \text{ gtt}$$
$$x = 20 \times 1{,}000$$
$$x = 20{,}000 \text{ gtt}$$

Step 2: Calculate required minutes.

$$500 \text{ U} : 60 \text{ min} :: 10{,}000 \text{ U} : x \text{ min}$$
$$500x = 60 \times 10{,}000$$
$$x = \frac{600{,}000}{500}$$
$$x = 1{,}200 \text{ minutes}$$

Step 3: Calculate the flow rate.

$$1{,}200 \text{ min} : 20{,}000 \text{ gtt} :: 1 \text{ min} : x \text{ gtt}$$
$$1{,}200x = 20{,}000$$
$$x = \frac{20{,}000}{1{,}200}$$
$$x = 16.6 \text{ or } 17 \text{ gtt/minute}$$

74 Correct answer — **A**

D/A

$$\frac{10 \, \cancel{mU}}{1 \text{ min}} \times \frac{\overset{1}{\cancel{500}} \, \cancel{ml}}{\underset{10}{\cancel{5{,}000}} \, \cancel{mU}} \times \frac{15 \text{ gtt}}{1 \, \cancel{ml}} = \frac{150 \text{ gtt}}{10 \text{ min}} = 15 \text{ gtt/minute}$$

R/P

Step 1: Change milliliters to drops.

$$1 \text{ ml} : 15 \text{ gtt} :: 500 \text{ ml} : x \text{ gtt}$$
$$x = 15 \times 500$$
$$x = 7{,}500 \text{ gtt}$$

Step 2: Calculate required minutes.

$$10 \text{ mU} : 1 \text{ min} :: 5{,}000 \text{ mU} : x \text{ min}$$
$$10x = 5{,}000$$
$$x = \frac{5{,}000}{10}$$
$$x = 500 \text{ minutes}$$

Step 3: Calculate the flow rate.

$$500 \text{ min} : 7{,}500 \text{ gtt} :: 1 \text{ min} : x \text{ gtt}$$
$$500x = 7{,}500$$
$$x = \frac{7{,}500}{500}$$
$$x = 15 \text{ gtt/minute}$$

75 Correct answer — **B**

D/A

$$\frac{\overset{1}{\cancel{15}} \text{ }\cancel{mg}}{\underset{3}{\cancel{60}} \text{ min}} \times \frac{500 \text{ }\cancel{ml}}{\underset{5}{\cancel{75}} \text{ }\cancel{mg}} \times \frac{\overset{1}{\cancel{20}} \text{ gtt}}{1 \text{ }\cancel{ml}} = \frac{500 \text{ gtt}}{15 \text{ min}} = 33.3 \text{ or } 33 \text{ gtt/minute}$$

R/P

Step 1: Change milliliters to drops.

$$1 \text{ ml} : 20 \text{ gtt} :: 500 \text{ ml} : x \text{ gtt}$$
$$x = 20 \times 500$$
$$x = 10{,}000 \text{ gtt}$$

Step 2: Calculate required minutes.

$$15 \text{ mg} : 60 \text{ min} :: 75 \text{ mg} : x \text{ min}$$
$$15x = 60 \times 75$$
$$x = \frac{4{,}500}{15}$$
$$x = 300 \text{ minutes}$$

Step 3: Calculate the flow rate.

$$300 \text{ min} : 10{,}000 \text{ gtt} :: 1 \text{ min} : x \text{ gtt}$$
$$300x = 10{,}000$$
$$x = \frac{10{,}000}{300}$$
$$x = 33.3 \text{ or } 33 \text{ gtt/minute}$$

76 Correct answer — **D**

D/A

$$\frac{0.04 \text{ mg}}{1 \text{ min}} \times \frac{500 \text{ ml}}{\underset{1}{\cancel{2} \text{ mg}}} \times \frac{\overset{5}{\cancel{10} \text{ gtt}}}{1 \text{ ml}} = 100 \text{ gtt/minute}$$

R/P

Step 1: Change milliliters to drops.
$$1 \text{ ml} : 10 \text{ gtt} :: 500 \text{ ml} : x \text{ gtt}$$
$$x = 10 \times 500$$
$$x = 5,000 \text{ gtt}$$

Step 2: Calculate required minutes.
$$0.04 \text{ mg} : 1 \text{ min} :: 2 \text{ mg} : x \text{ min}$$
$$0.04x = 2$$
$$x = \frac{2}{0.04}$$
$$x = 50 \text{ minutes}$$

Step 3: Calculate the flow rate.
$$50 \text{ min} : 5,000 \text{ gtt} :: 1 \text{ min} : x \text{ gtt}$$
$$50x = 5,000$$
$$x = \frac{5,000}{50}$$
$$x = 100 \text{ gtt/minute}$$

77 Correct answer — **B**

D/A

$$\frac{1 \text{ mg}}{1 \text{ min}} \times \frac{\overset{10}{\cancel{1,000} \text{ ml}}}{\underset{12}{\cancel{1,200} \text{ mg}}} \times \frac{60 \text{ mcgtt}}{1 \text{ ml}} = \frac{600 \text{ mcgtt}}{12 \text{ min}} = 50 \text{ mcgtt/minute}$$

R/P

Step 1: Change milliliters to microdrops.
$$1 \text{ ml} : 60 \text{ mcgtt} :: 1,000 \text{ ml} : x \text{ mcgtt}$$
$$x = 60 \times 1,000$$
$$x = 60,000 \text{ mcgtt}$$

Step 2: Calculate required minutes.
$$1 \text{ mg} : 1 \text{ min} :: 1,200 \text{ mg} : x \text{ min}$$
$$x = 1,200 \text{ minutes}$$

Step 3: Calculate the flow rate.

1,200 min : 60,000 mcgtt :: 1 min : x mcgtt

$$1,200x = 60,000$$

$$x = \frac{60,000}{1,200}$$

$$x = 50 \text{ mcgtt/minute}$$

78 Correct answer—A

D/A

$$\frac{\overset{1}{\cancel{25,000\,U}}}{1 \text{ min}} \times \frac{100 \cancel{\text{ml}}}{\underset{120}{\cancel{3,000,000\,U}}} \times \frac{15 \text{ gtt}}{1 \cancel{\text{ml}}} =$$

$$\frac{1,500 \text{ gtt}}{120 \text{ min}} = 12.5 \text{ or } 13 \text{ gtt/minute}$$

R/P

Step 1: Change milliliters to drops.

1 ml : 15 gtt :: 100 ml : x gtt

$$x = 15 \times 100$$

$$x = 1,500 \text{ gtt}$$

Step 2: Calculate required minutes.

25,000 U : 1 min :: 3,000,000 U : x min

$$25,000x = 3,000,000$$

$$x = \frac{3,000,000}{25,000}$$

$$x = 120 \text{ minutes}$$

Step 3: Calculate the flow rate.

120 min : 1,500 gtt :: 1 min : x gtt

$$120x = 1,500$$

$$x = \frac{1,500}{120}$$

$$x = 12.5 \text{ or } 13 \text{ gtt/minute}$$

79 Correct answer—C

D/A

$$\frac{15 \cancel{\text{mg}}}{1 \text{ min}} \times \frac{\overset{1}{\cancel{100}}\cancel{\text{ml}}}{\underset{3}{\cancel{300}}\cancel{\text{mg}}} \times \frac{10 \text{ gtt}}{1 \cancel{\text{ml}}} = \frac{150 \text{ gtt}}{3 \text{ min}} = 50 \text{ gtt/minute}$$

R/P

Step 1: Change milliliters to drops.

$$1 \text{ ml} : 10 \text{ gtt} :: 100 \text{ ml} : x \text{ gtt}$$
$$x = 10 \times 100$$
$$x = 1{,}000 \text{ gtt}$$

Step 2: Calculate required minutes.

$$15 \text{ mg} : 1 \text{ min} :: 300 \text{ mg} : x \text{ min}$$
$$15x = 300$$
$$x = \frac{300}{15}$$
$$x = 20 \text{ minutes}$$

Step 3: Calculate the flow rate.

$$20 \text{ min} : 1{,}000 \text{ gtt} :: 1 \text{ min} : x \text{ gtt}$$
$$20x = 1{,}000$$
$$x = \frac{1{,}000}{20}$$
$$x = 50 \text{ gtt/minute}$$

80 Correct answer — **A**

D/A

$$\frac{0.22 \text{ mg}}{1 \text{ min}} \times \frac{\overset{4}{1{,}000} \text{ ml}}{\underset{1}{250} \text{ mg}} \times \frac{15 \text{ gtt}}{1 \text{ ml}} = 13.2 \text{ or } 13 \text{ gtt/minute}$$

R/P

Step 1: Change milliliters to drops.

$$1 \text{ ml} : 15 \text{ gtt} :: 1{,}000 \text{ ml} : x \text{ gtt}$$
$$x = 15{,}000 \text{ gtt}$$

Step 2: Calculate required minutes.

$$0.22 \text{ mg} : 1 \text{ min} :: 250 \text{ mg} : x \text{ min}$$
$$0.22x = 250$$
$$x = \frac{250}{0.22}$$
$$x = 1{,}136 \text{ minutes}$$

Step 3: Calculate the flow rate.

$$1{,}136 \text{ min} : 15{,}000 \text{ gtt} :: 1 \text{ min} : x \text{ gtt}$$
$$1{,}136x = 15{,}000$$
$$x = \frac{15{,}000}{1{,}136}$$
$$x = 13.2 \text{ or } 13 \text{ gtt/minute}$$

81 Correct answer—C

Remember: 0.5 g = 500 mg

D/A

$$\frac{2.6 \text{ mg}}{1 \text{ min}} \times \frac{\overset{1}{\cancel{250}} \text{ ml}}{\underset{2}{\cancel{500}} \text{ mg}} \times \frac{60 \text{ mcgtt}}{1 \text{ ml}} = \frac{156 \text{ mcgtt}}{2 \text{ min}} = 78 \text{ mcgtt/minute}$$

R/P

Step 1: Change milliliters to microdrops.

$$1 \text{ ml} : 60 \text{ mcgtt} :: 250 \text{ ml} : x \text{ mcgtt}$$
$$x = 60 \times 250$$
$$x = 15,000 \text{ mcgtt}$$

Step 2: Calculate required minutes.

$$2.6 \text{ mg} : 1 \text{ min} :: 500 \text{ mg} : x \text{ min}$$
$$2.6x = 500$$
$$x = \frac{500}{2.6}$$
$$x = 192.3 \text{ minutes}$$

Step 3: Calculate the flow rate.

$$192.3 \text{ min} : 15,000 \text{ mcgtt} :: 1 \text{ min} : x \text{ mcgtt}$$
$$192.3x = 15,000$$
$$x = \frac{15,000}{192.3}$$
$$x = 78 \text{ mcgtt/minute}$$

82 Correct answer—B

Remember: 1 U = 1,000 mU

D/A

$$\frac{12.5 \text{ mU}}{1 \text{ min}} \times \frac{\overset{75}{\cancel{750}} \text{ ml}}{\underset{1,000}{\cancel{10,000}} \text{ mU}} \times \frac{15 \text{ gtt}}{1 \text{ ml}} = \frac{14,062.5 \text{ gtt}}{1,000 \text{ min}} = 14 \text{ gtt/minute}$$

R/P

Step 1: Change milliliters to drops.

$$1 \text{ ml} : 15 \text{ gtt} :: 750 \text{ ml} : x \text{ gtt}$$
$$x = 15 \times 750$$
$$x = 11,250 \text{ gtt}$$

Step 2: Calculate required minutes.

$$12.5 \text{ mU} : 1 \text{ min} :: 10,000 \text{ mU} : x \text{ min}$$
$$12.5x = 10,000$$
$$x = \frac{10,000}{12.5}$$
$$x = 800 \text{ minutes}$$

Step 3: Calculate the flow rate.

800 min : 11,250 gtt :: 1 min : x gtt

$$800x = 11,250$$

$$x = \frac{11,250}{800}$$

$$x = 14 \text{ gtt/minute}$$

83 Correct answer — **C**

D/A

$$\frac{7.5 \ \overset{}{\text{m\!Eq}}}{\underset{1}{\cancel{60} \ \text{min}}} \times \frac{\overset{10}{\cancel{250} \ \cancel{\text{ml}}}}{\underset{1}{\cancel{25} \ \cancel{\text{m\!Eq}}}} \times \frac{\overset{1}{\cancel{60} \ \text{mcgtt}}}{1 \ \cancel{\text{ml}}} = 75 \text{ mcgtt/minute}$$

R/P

Step 1: Change milliliters to microdrops.

1 ml : 60 mcgtt :: 250 ml : x mcgtt

$$x = 60 \times 250$$

$$x = 15,000 \text{ mcgtt}$$

Step 2: Calculate required minutes.

7.5 mEq : 60 min :: 25 mEq : x min

$$7.5x = 60 \times 25$$

$$x = \frac{1,500}{7.5}$$

$$x = 200 \text{ minutes}$$

Step 3: Calculate the flow rate.

200 min : 15,000 mcgtt :: 1 min : x mcgtt

$$200x = 15,000$$

$$x = \frac{15,000}{200}$$

$$x = 75 \text{ mcgtt/minute}$$

84 Correct answer — **A**

D/A

$$50 \ \cancel{\text{kg}} \times \frac{0.005 \ \cancel{\text{mg/kg}}}{\text{min}} \times \frac{\overset{1}{\cancel{250} \ \cancel{\text{ml}}}}{\underset{1}{\cancel{250} \ \cancel{\text{mg}}}} \times \frac{60 \ \text{mcgtt}}{1 \ \cancel{\text{ml}}} = 15 \text{ mcgtt/minute}$$

R/P

Step 1: Change milliliters to microdrops.
$$1 \text{ ml} : 60 \text{ mcgtt} :: 250 \text{ ml} : x \text{ mcgtt}$$
$$x = 60 \times 250$$
$$x = 15{,}000 \text{ mcgtt}$$

Step 2: Calculate the number of milligrams per minute.
$$1 \text{ kg} : 0.005 \text{ mg/min} :: 50 \text{ kg} : x \text{ mg/min}$$
$$x = 0.005 \times 50$$
$$x = 0.25 \text{ mg/minute}$$

Step 3: Calculate required minutes.
$$0.25 \text{ mg} : 1 \text{ min} :: 250 \text{ mg} : x \text{ min}$$
$$0.25x = 250$$
$$x = \frac{250}{0.25}$$
$$x = 1{,}000 \text{ minutes}$$

Step 4: Calculate the flow rate.
$$1{,}000 \text{ min} : 15{,}000 \text{ mcgtt} :: 1 \text{ min} : x \text{ mcgtt}$$
$$1{,}000x = 15{,}000$$
$$x = \frac{15{,}000}{1{,}000}$$
$$x = 15 \text{ mcgtt/minute}$$

85 Correct answer — **B**

D/A

$$72 \ \cancel{\text{kg}} \times \frac{0.01 \ \cancel{\text{mg/kg}}}{\text{min}} \times \frac{\overset{5}{\cancel{500}} \ \cancel{\text{ml}}}{\underset{4}{\cancel{400}} \ \cancel{\text{mg}}} \times \frac{60 \text{ mcgtt}}{1 \ \cancel{\text{ml}}} =$$

$$\frac{216 \text{ mcgtt}}{4 \text{ min}} = 54 \text{ mcgtt/minute}$$

R/P

Step 1: Change milliliters to microdrops.
$$1 \text{ ml} : 60 \text{ mcgtt} :: 500 \text{ ml} : x \text{ mcgtt}$$
$$x = 60 \times 500$$
$$x = 30{,}000 \text{ mcgtt}$$

Step 2: Calculate the number of milligrams per minute.
$$1 \text{ kg} : 0.01 \text{ mg/min} :: 72 \text{ kg} : x \text{ mg/min}$$
$$x = 0.01 \times 72$$
$$x = 0.72 \text{ mg/minute}$$

Step 3: Calculate required minutes.
$$0.72 \text{ mg} : 1 \text{ min} :: 400 \text{ mg} : x \text{ min}$$
$$0.72x = 400$$
$$x = \frac{400}{0.72}$$
$$x = 555.5 \text{ minutes}$$

Step 4: Calculate the flow rate.
$$555.5 \text{ min} : 30,000 \text{ mcgtt} :: 1 \text{ min} : x \text{ mcgtt}$$
$$555.5x = 30,000$$
$$x = \frac{30,000}{555.5}$$
$$x = 54 \text{ mcgtt/minute}$$

86 Correct answer — C

D/A

$$65 \ \cancel{\text{kg}} \times \frac{0.008 \ \cancel{\text{mg/kg}}}{\text{min}} \times \frac{\overset{10}{\cancel{500}} \ \cancel{\text{ml}}}{\underset{7}{\cancel{350}} \ \cancel{\text{mg}}} \times \frac{60 \ \text{mcgtt}}{1 \ \cancel{\text{ml}}} =$$

$$\frac{312 \ \text{mcgtt}}{7 \ \text{min}} = 44.5 \text{ or } 45 \text{ mcgtt/minute}$$

R/P

Step 1: Change milliliters to microdrops.
$$1 \text{ ml} : 60 \text{ mcgtt} :: 500 \text{ ml} : x \text{ mcgtt}$$
$$x = 60 \times 500$$
$$x = 30,000 \text{ mcgtt}$$

Step 2: Calculate the number of milligrams per minute.
$$1 \text{ kg} : 0.008 \text{ mg/min} :: 65 \text{ kg} : x \text{ mg/min}$$
$$x = 0.008 \times 65$$
$$x = 0.52 \text{ mg/minute}$$

Step 3: Calculate required minutes.
$$0.52 \text{ mg} : 1 \text{ min} :: 350 \text{ mg} : x \text{ min}$$
$$0.52x = 350 \text{ mg}$$
$$x = \frac{350}{0.52}$$
$$x = 673 \text{ minutes}$$

Step 4: Calculate the flow rate.
$$673 \text{ min} : 30,000 \text{ mcgtt} :: 1 \text{ min} : x \text{ mcgtt}$$
$$673x = 30,000$$
$$x = \frac{30,000}{673}$$
$$x = 44.5 \text{ or } 45 \text{ mcgtt/minute}$$

87 Correct answer — C

D/A

$$50 \text{ kg} \times \frac{4{,}400 \text{ U/kg}}{\text{hr}} \times \frac{\overset{1}{1{,}000 \text{ ml}}}{\underset{2{,}500}{2{,}500{,}000 \text{ U}}} \times \frac{15 \text{ gtt}}{1 \text{ ml}} \times \frac{1 \text{ hr}}{60 \text{ min}} =$$

$$\frac{330{,}000 \text{ gtt}}{15{,}000 \text{ min}} = 22 \text{ gtt/minute}$$

R/P

Step 1: Change milliliters to drops.
$$1 \text{ ml} : 15 \text{ gtt} :: 1{,}000 \text{ ml} : x \text{ gtt}$$
$$x = 15 \times 1{,}000$$
$$x = 15{,}000 \text{ gtt}$$

Step 2: Calculate the number of units per minute.
$$1 \text{ kg} : 4{,}400 \text{ U/hr} :: 50 \text{ kg} : x \text{ U/hr}$$
$$x = 4{,}400 \times 50$$
$$x = 220{,}000 \text{ U/hr}$$
$$220{,}000 \text{ U/hour} = 3{,}666.6 \text{ U/minute}$$

Step 3: Calculate required minutes
$$3{,}666.6 \text{ U} : 1 \text{ min} :: 2{,}500{,}000 \text{ U} : x \text{ min}$$
$$3{,}666.6x = 2{,}500{,}000$$
$$x = \frac{2{,}500{,}000}{3{,}666.6}$$
$$x = 681.8 \text{ minutes}$$

Step 4: Calculate the flow rate.
$$681.8 \text{ min} : 15{,}000 \text{ gtt} :: 1 \text{ min} : x \text{ gtt}$$
$$681.8x = 15{,}000$$
$$x = \frac{15{,}000}{681.8}$$
$$x = 22 \text{ gtt/minute}$$

88 Correct answer — A

Remember: 1 mg = 1,000 mcg

D/A

$$70 \text{ kg} \times \frac{0.5 \text{ mcg/kg}}{\text{min}} \times \frac{\overset{1}{250 \text{ ml}}}{\underset{200}{50{,}000 \text{ mcg}}} \times \frac{60 \text{ mcgtt}}{1 \text{ ml}} =$$

$$\frac{2{,}100 \text{ mcgtt}}{200 \text{ min}} = 10.5 \text{ or } 11 \text{ mcgtt/minute}$$

R/P

Step 1: Change milliliters to microdrops.
$$1 \text{ ml} : 60 \text{ mcgtt} :: 250 \text{ ml} : x \text{ mcgtt}$$
$$x = 60 \times 250$$
$$x = 15,000 \text{ mcgtt}$$

Step 2: Calculate the number of micrograms per minute.
$$1 \text{ kg} : 0.5 \text{ mcg/min} :: 70 \text{ kg} : x \text{ mcg/min}$$
$$x = 0.5 \times 70$$
$$x = 35 \text{ mcg/minute}$$

Step 3: Calculate required minutes.
$$35 \text{ mcg} : 1 \text{ min} :: 50,000 \text{ mcg} : x \text{ min}$$
$$35x = 50,000$$
$$x = \frac{50,000}{35}$$
$$x = 1,428.5 \text{ minute}$$

Step 4: Calculate the flow rate.
$$1,428.5 \text{ min} : 15,000 \text{ mcgtt} :: 1 \text{ min} : x \text{ mcgtt}$$
$$1,428.5x = 15,000$$
$$x = \frac{15,000}{1,428.5}$$
$$x = 10.5 \text{ or } 11 \text{ mcgtt/minute}$$

CHAPTER 8

Complex Calculations

Questions

1 The nurse administers a dopamine (Intropin) infusion to a 70-kg patient, as ordered. The solution, which consists of 500 mg of dopamine added to 250 ml of dextrose 5% in water (D_5W), is administered at a flow rate of 21 mcgtt/minute using a microdrop setup (60 mcgtt = 1 ml). How many micrograms per kilogram per minute is the patient receiving?

A. 5 mcg/kg/minute
B. 10 mcg/kg/minute
C. 20 mcg/kg/minute
D. 25 mcg/kg/minute

2 A patient weighing 55 kg is receiving an infusion of 500 mg of dobutamine (Dobutrex) in 250 ml of D_5W at a rate of 10 ml/hour. How many micrograms per kilogram per minute of this inotropic medication is the patient receiving?

A. 4 mcg/kg/minute
B. 5 mcg/kg/minute
C. 6 mcg/kg/minute
D. 8 mcg/kg/minute

3 A 45-kg patient is scheduled to receive 500 mg of the antihypertensive drug trimethaphan (Arfonad) in 500 ml of D_5W. The physician has ordered the infusion to run at a rate of 45 ml/hour. How many micrograms per kilogram per hour will this patient receive?

A. 10 mcg/kg/hour
B. 100 mcg/kg/hour
C. 500 mcg/kg/hour
D. 1,000 mcg/kg/hour

SITUATION

The nurse prepares an infusion of 100 mg of the coronary vasodilator nitroglycerin (Nitro-Bid I.V.) in 500 ml of D_5W for a patient weighing 40 kg. The physician's order stipulates that the infusion should run at a rate of 25 mcgtt/minute.

Questions 4 and 5 refer to this situation.

4 How many milligrams per kilogram per minute would the patient receive?

A. 0.0004 mg/kg/minute
B. 0.0008 mg/kg/minute
C. 0.002 mg/kg/minute
D. 0.95 mg/kg/minute

5 How many micrograms per kilogram per minute will the patient receive?

A. 0.04 mcg/kg/minute
B. 0.2 mcg/kg/minute
C. 0.8 mcg/kg/minute
D. 2 mcg/kg/minute

SITUATION

A 50-kg patient is receiving an infusion of 250 ml of D$_5$W with 100 mg of nitroglycerin at a rate of 12 ml/hour.

Questions 6 and 7 refer to this situation.

6 How many micrograms per kilogram per minute of this coronary vasodilator is the patient receiving?

A. 1 mcg/kg/minute
B. 1.6 mcg/kg/minute
C. 12 mcg/kg/minute
D. 100 mcg/kg/minute

7 How many milligrams per kilogram per minute is this patient receiving?

A. 0.0004 mg/kg/minute
B. 0.0008 mg/kg/minute
C. 0.0016 mg/kg/minute
D. 0.125 mg/kg/minute

SITUATION

A patient weighing 60 kg is receiving an infusion of 250 ml of D$_5$W with 50 mg of the vasopressor nitroprusside (Nipride). The solution is infusing at a rate of 20 ml/hour.

Questions 8 and 9 refer to this situation.

8 How many milligrams per kilogram per hour is the patient receiving?

A. 0.003 mg/kg/hour
B. 0.066 mg/kg/hour
C. 3 mg/kg/hour
D. 12.4 mg/kg/hour

9 What is the equivalent in micrograms per kilogram per minute?

A. 1.1 mcg/kg/minute
B. 10.5 mcg/kg/minute
C. 14 mcg/kg/minute
D. 60 mcg/kg/minute

SITUATION

A patient weighing 70 kg is receiving 16 U of regular insulin per hour from an I.V. solution of 250 ml of normal saline solution that contains 100 U of insulin.

Questions 10 and 11 refer to this situation.

10 How many milliliters per hour are being infused?

A. 40 ml/hour
B. 49 ml/hour
C. 82 ml/hour
D. 99.1 ml/hour

11 How many units per kilogram per minute is the patient receiving?

A. 0.0007 U/kg/minute
B. 0.004 U/kg/minute
C. 0.1 U/kg/minute
D. 3 U/kg/minute

SITUATION

The nurse adds 100 U of insulin to 250 ml of normal saline solution.

Questions 12 and 13 refer to this situation.

12 What is the insulin concentration of this solution?

A. 1:2
B. 1:4
C. 2:3
D. 2:5

13 What is the percent strength of the solution?

A. 20%
B. 40%
C. 50%
D. 60%

SITUATION

The physician's order for a 70-kg patient receiving an infusion of D_5W reads: "Administer 250 mg of dopamine (Intropin) in 250 ml of D_5W at a rate of 166.6 mcg/minute."

Questions 14 and 15 refer to this situation.

14 How many milliliters of this solution will the patient receive in 24 hours?

A. 24 ml
B. 48 ml
C. 180 ml
D. 240 ml

15 The physician changes the order to read "Give 500 mg of dopamine in 500 ml of D_5W at a rate of 3.6 mcg/kg/minute." What is the current flow rate in milliliters per hour?

A. 12 ml/hour
B. 15 ml/hour
C. 30 ml/hour
D. 45 ml/hour

SITUATION

The physician orders the following: an intravenous piggyback (IVPB) infusion of cefazolin (Ancef) 1 mg in 100 ml D$_5$W to infuse over 60 minutes q4h; an IVPB of metronidazole (Flagyl) 500 mg in 50 ml D$_5$W over 30 minutes q6h; an infusion of heparin 12,500 U in 250 ml D$_5$W at a rate of 500 U/hour via a central line.

Questions 16 and 17 refer to this situation.

16 What is the flow rate, in microdrops per minute, for each of the drugs infused?

A. Cefazolin, 10 mcgtt/minute; metronidazole, 50 mcgtt/minute; heparin, 100 mcgtt/minute
B. Cefazolin, 100 mcgtt/minute; metronidazole, 10 mcgtt/minute; heparin, 25 mcgtt/minute
C. Cefazolin 100 mcgtt/minute; metronidazole, 100 mcgtt/minute; heparin, 10 mcgtt/minute
D. Cefazolin 100 mcgtt/minute; metronidazole, 10 mcgtt/minute; heparin, 100 mcgtt/minute

17 If the patient is to receive a total of 2,400 ml of I.V. solution in 24 hours, what would be the infusion rate (in microdrops per minute) of the primary-line solution of dextrose 5% in ½ normal saline?

A. 20 mcgtt/minute
B. 40 mcgtt/minute
C. 75 mcgtt/minute
D. 85 mcgtt/minute

SITUATION

The nurse notes on the patient's chart that he is to receive dimethyl sulfoxide (Demasorb), which is primarily ordered for symptomatic relief of interstitial cystitis. The drug is supplied in vials labeled 50% in 50 ml.

Questions 18 and 19 refer to this situation.

18 If 50 ml are instilled in the urinary bladder, how many grams will the patient receive?

A. 25 g
B. 40 g
C. 50 g
D. 60 g

19 If 50 ml of the 50% solution are added to 450 ml of sterile water, what will be the percent concentration of the total solution?

A. 2%
B. 5%
C. 10%
D. 20%

SITUATION

A physician plans to give a 75-kg patient scheduled for hip surgery low molecular weight dextran (Dextran 40) as a plasma expander. The usual order is 10 ml/kg I.V.

Questions 20 to 22 refer to this situation.

20 This drug is supplied in 500-ml containers; how many milliliters must the patient receive?

A. 100 ml
B. 380 ml
C. 600 ml
D. 750 ml

21 How many milliliters per hour will the patient receive if the total amount must be infused in 24 hours?

A. 12 ml/hour
B. 31 ml/hour
C. 42 ml/hour
D. 60 ml/hour

22 What is the flow rate if the drop factor is 10 gtt = 1 ml?

A. 1 gtt/minute
B. 5 gtt/minute
C. 10 gtt/minute
D. 16 gtt/minute

SITUATION

A patient has had abdominal surgery and is in the postanesthesia care unit. The physician orders doxapram hydrochloride (Dopram), a postoperative respiratory stimulant, 5 mg/minute for 10 minutes, followed by 3 mg/minute for 20 minutes, then 1 mg/minute for 30 minutes.

Questions 23 and 24 refer to this situation.

23 What is the flow rate for each dosage ordered if 400 mg of doxapram are added to 250 ml of D_5W and the drop factor is 10 gtt = 1 ml?

A. 1 gtt/minute, 3 gtt/minute, 7 gtt/minute
B. 10 gtt/minute, 3 gtt/minute, 1 gtt/minute
C. 31 gtt/minute, 19 gtt/minute, 6 gtt/minute
D. 64 gtt/minute, 29 gtt/minute, 12 gtt/minute

24 How much I.V. solution will the patient receive in 1 hour?

A. 28 ml
B. 40 ml
C. 70.4 ml
D. 87 ml

SITUATION

The physician writes the following order for a patient who weighs 40 kg: 250 ml of D_5W with 800 mg dopamine (Intropin) at 5 ml/hour via a central line (60 mcgtt = 1 ml); 700 ml packed red blood cells IVPB over 4 hours; and a KVO I.V. solution of normal saline via a primary line (10 gtt = 1 ml).

Questions 25 and 26 refer to this situation.

25 How many micrograms per kilogram per minute will the patient receive by the central line?

A. 2 mcg/kg/minute
B. 6.6 mcg/kg/minute
C. 13 mcg/kg/minute
D. 23 mcg/kg/minute

26 If the patient's total intake is restricted to 1,500 ml/24 hours, what will be the flow rate for the KVO infusion?

A. 6 gtt/minute
B. 10 gtt/minute
C. 11.5 gtt/minute
D. 62 gtt/minute

SITUATION

A 50-kg patient is currently receiving 250 ml of D$_5$W with 500 mg of lidocaine (Xylocaine), an antiarrhythmic, at 150 mcgtt/minute.

Questions 27 and 28 refer to this situation.

27 How many milligrams per kilogram per minute of this I.V. solution would the patient receive?

A. 0.04 mg/kg/minute
B. 0.1 mg/kg/minute
C. 1.7 mg/kg/minute
D. 2.2 mg/kg/minute

28 If the I.V. infusion were decreased to a rate of 4 mcg/kg/minute, what would the equivalent flow rate be in microdrops per minute?

A. 2 mcgtt/minute
B. 3 mcgtt/minute
C. 6 mcgtt/minute
D. 12 mcgtt/minute

SITUATION

A patient is to receive 250 ml of normal saline solution with 50 U of regular insulin (Humulin R) at a flow rate of 18 gtt/minute. The drop factor is 10 gtt = 1 ml.

Questions 29 to 31 refer to this situation.

29 How many units of this solution will the patient receive per hour?

A. 21.6 U/hour
B. 25 U/hour
C. 49 U/hour
D. 53 U/hour

30 How long will the infusion last?

A. 1 hour, 4 minutes
B. 1 hour, 53 minutes
C. 2 hours, 6 minutes
D. 2 hours, 18 minutes

31 What is the percent concentration of the solution?

A. 10%
B. 20%
C. 30%
D. 50%

Answer sheet

	A	B	C	D		A	B	C	D
1	○	○	○	○	31	○	○	○	○
2	○	○	○	○					
3	○	○	○	○					
4	○	○	○	○					
5	○	○	○	○					
6	○	○	○	○					
7	○	○	○	○					
8	○	○	○	○					
9	○	○	○	○					
10	○	○	○	○					
11	○	○	○	○					
12	○	○	○	○					
13	○	○	○	○					
14	○	○	○	○					
15	○	○	○	○					
16	○	○	○	○					
17	○	○	○	○					
18	○	○	○	○					
19	○	○	○	○					
20	○	○	○	○					
21	○	○	○	○					
22	○	○	○	○					
23	○	○	○	○					
24	○	○	○	○					
25	○	○	○	○					
26	○	○	○	○					
27	○	○	○	○					
28	○	○	○	○					
29	○	○	○	○					
30	○	○	○	○					

Answers

1 Correct answer — **B**

D/A

$$\frac{21 \text{ mcgtt}}{70 \text{ kg/min}} \times \frac{1 \text{ ml}}{\underset{6}{60} \text{ mcgtt}} \times \frac{\overset{50}{500} \text{ mg}}{\underset{1}{250} \text{ ml}} \times \frac{\overset{4}{1{,}000} \text{ mcg}}{1 \text{ mg}} =$$

$$\frac{4{,}200 \text{ mcg}}{420 \text{ kg/minute}} = 10 \text{ mcg/kg/minute}$$

R/P

Step 1: Change milliliters to microdrops.

$$1 \text{ ml} : 60 \text{ mcgtt} :: 250 \text{ ml} : x \text{ mcgtt}$$
$$x = 60 \times 250$$
$$x = 15{,}000 \text{ mcgtt}$$

Step 2: Calculate milligrams administered in a minute.

$$15{,}000 \text{ mcgtt} : 500 \text{ mg} :: 21 \text{ mcgtt} : x \text{ mg}$$
$$15{,}000x = 500 \times 21$$
$$x = \frac{10{,}500}{15{,}000}$$
$$x = 0.7 \text{ mg}$$

Step 3: Change milligrams to micrograms.

$$1 \text{ mg} : 1{,}000 \text{ mcg} :: 0.7 \text{ mg} : x \text{ mcg}$$
$$x = 1{,}000 \times 0.7$$
$$x = 700 \text{ mcg}$$

Step 4: Calculate micrograms per kilogram per minute.

$$70 \text{ kg} : 700 \text{ mcg} :: 1 \text{ kg} : x \text{ mg}$$
$$70x = 700$$
$$x = \frac{700}{70}$$
$$x = 10 \text{ mcg/kg/minute}$$

2 Correct answer — **C**

D/A

$$\frac{\overset{1}{10} \text{ ml}}{\underset{6}{55} \text{ kg/60 min}} \times \frac{\overset{}{500} \text{ mg}}{\underset{1}{250} \text{ ml}} \times \frac{\overset{4}{1{,}000} \text{ mcg}}{1 \text{ mg}} =$$

$$\frac{2{,}000 \text{ mcg}}{330 \text{ kg/min}} = 6 \text{ mcg/kg/minute}$$

R/P

Step 1: Calculate milligrams administered in an hour.

$$250 \text{ ml} : 500 \text{ mg} :: 10 \text{ ml} : x \text{ mg}$$
$$250x = 500 \times 10$$
$$x = \frac{5{,}000}{250}$$
$$x = 20 \text{ mg}$$

Step 2: Change milligrams to micrograms

$$1 \text{ mg} : 1{,}000 \text{ mcg} :: 20 \text{ mg} : x \text{ mcg}$$
$$x = 1{,}000 \times 20$$
$$x = 20{,}000 \text{ mcg}$$

Step 3: Calculate micrograms administered in a minute.

$$60 \text{ min} : 20{,}000 \text{ mcg} :: 1 \text{ min} : x \text{ mcg}$$
$$60x = 20{,}000$$
$$x = \frac{20{,}000}{60}$$
$$x = 333.3 \text{ mcg}$$

Step 4: Calculate micrograms per kilogram per minute.

$$55 \text{ kg} : 333.3 \text{ mcg} :: 1 \text{ kg} : x \text{ mcg}$$
$$55x = 333.3$$
$$x = \frac{333.3}{55}$$
$$x = 6 \text{ mcg/kg/minute}$$

3 Correct answer — **D**

D/A

$$\frac{\overset{1}{\cancel{45} \text{ ml}}}{\underset{1}{\cancel{45} \text{ kg/hr}}} \times \frac{\overset{1}{\cancel{500} \text{ mg}}}{\underset{1}{\cancel{500} \text{ ml}}} \times \frac{1{,}000 \text{ mcg}}{1 \cancel{\text{ mg}}} = 1{,}000 \text{ mcg/kg/hour}$$

R/P

Step 1: Calculate milligrams in a milliliter.

$$500 \text{ ml} : 500 \text{ mg} :: 1 \text{ ml} : x \text{ mg}$$
$$x = 1 \text{ mg}$$

Step 2: Calculate milligrams administered in an hour.

$$1 \text{ ml} : 1 \text{ mg} :: 45 \text{ ml} : x \text{ mg}$$
$$x = 45 \text{ mg}$$

Step 3: Calculate milligrams per kilogram per hour.

$$45 \text{ kg} : 45 \text{ mg} :: 1 \text{ kg} : x \text{ mg}$$
$$x = 1 \text{ mg/kg/hour}$$

Step 4: Calculate micrograms per kilogram per hour.

Because 1 mg = 1,000 mcg, the patient is receiving 1,000 mcg/kg/hour.

4 Correct answer — **C**

D/A

$$\frac{\overset{5}{\cancel{25}}\text{ mcgtt}}{\underset{8}{\cancel{40}}\text{ kg/min}} \times \frac{1\text{ } \cancel{\text{ml}}}{60\text{ mcgtt}} \times \frac{\overset{1}{\cancel{100}}\text{ mg}}{\underset{5}{\cancel{500}}\text{ } \cancel{\text{ml}}} =$$

$$\frac{5\text{ mg}}{2,400\text{ kg/min}} = 0.002\text{ mg/kg/minute}$$

R/P

Step 1: Change milliliters to microdrops.
$$1\text{ ml} : 60\text{ mcgtt} :: 500\text{ ml} : x\text{ mcgtt}$$
$$x = 60 \times 500$$
$$x = 30,000\text{ mcgtt}$$

Step 2: Calculate milligrams administered in a minute.
$$30,000\text{ mcgtt} : 100\text{ mg} :: 25\text{ mcgtt} : x\text{ mg}$$
$$30,000x = 100 \times 25$$
$$x = \frac{2,500}{30,000}$$
$$x = 0.083\text{ mg}$$

Step 3: Calculate milligrams per kilogram per minute.
$$40\text{ kg} : 0.083\text{ mg} :: 1\text{ kg} : x\text{ mg}$$
$$40x = 0.083$$
$$x = \frac{0.083}{40}$$
$$x = 0.002\text{ mg/kg/minute}$$

5 Correct answer — **D**

D/A

$$0.002\text{ } \cancel{\text{mg}}\text{/kg/min} \times \frac{1,000\text{ mcg}}{1\text{ } \cancel{\text{mg}}} = 2\text{ mcg/kg/minute}$$

R/P

$$1\text{ mg} : 1,000\text{ mcg} :: 0.002\text{ mg} : x\text{ mcg}$$
$$x = 1,000 \times 0.002$$
$$x = 2\text{ mcg/kg/minute}$$

6 Correct answer — **B**

D/A

$$\frac{12 \ \cancel{ml}}{\cancel{50} \ kg/60 \ min} \times \frac{\overset{2}{\cancel{100} \ \cancel{mg}}}{\cancel{250} \ \cancel{ml}} \times \frac{\overset{4}{1,000 \ mcg}}{1 \ \cancel{mg}} =$$

$$\frac{1 \qquad\qquad 1}{}$$

$$\frac{96 \ mcg}{60 \ kg/min} = 1.6 \ mcg/kg/minute$$

R/P

Step 1: Calculate milligrams administered in an hour.

$$250 \ ml : 100 \ mg :: 12 \ ml : x \ mg$$
$$250x = 100 \times 12$$
$$x = \frac{1,200}{250}$$
$$x = 4.8 \ mg$$

Step 2: Change milligrams to micrograms.

$$1 \ mg : 1,000 \ mcg :: 4.8 \ mg : x \ mcg$$
$$x = 1,000 \times 4.8$$
$$x = 4,800 \ mcg$$

Step 3: Determine the number of micrograms administered in a minute.

$$60 \ min : 4,800 \ mcg :: 1 \ min : x \ mcg$$
$$60x = 4,800$$
$$x = \frac{4,800}{60}$$
$$x = 80 \ mcg$$

Step 4: Calculate micrograms per kilogram per minute.

$$50 \ kg : 80 \ mcg :: 1 \ kg : x \ mcg$$
$$50x = 80$$
$$x = \frac{80}{50}$$
$$x = 1.6 \ mcg/kg/minute$$

7 Correct answer — **C**

D/A

$$\frac{1.6 \ \cancel{mcg}}{1 \ min} \times \frac{1 \ mg}{1,000 \ \cancel{mcg}} = \frac{1.6 \ mg}{1,000 \ min} = 0.0016 \ mg/kg/minute$$

R/P

$$1{,}000 \text{ mcg} : 1 \text{ mg} :: 1.6 \text{ mg} : x \text{ mcg}$$
$$1{,}000x = 1.6$$
$$x = \frac{1.6}{1{,}000}$$
$$x = 0.0016 \text{ mg/kg/minute}$$

---

8 Correct answer — **B**

D/A

$$\frac{\overset{1}{\cancel{20} \text{ ml}}}{\underset{3}{\cancel{60} \text{ kg/hr}}} \times \frac{\overset{1}{\cancel{50} \text{ mg}}}{\underset{5}{\cancel{250} \text{ ml}}} = \frac{1 \text{ mg}}{15 \text{ kg/hr}} = 0.066 \text{ mg/kg/hour}$$

R/P

Step 1: Calculate milligrams administered in an hour.
$$250 \text{ ml} : 50 \text{ mg} :: 20 \text{ ml} : x \text{ mg}$$
$$250x = 50 \times 20$$
$$x = \frac{1{,}000}{250}$$
$$x = 4 \text{ mg}$$

Step 2: Calculate milligrams per kilogram per hour.
$$60 \text{ kg} : 4 \text{ mg} :: 1 \text{ kg} : x \text{ mg}$$
$$4x = 60$$
$$x = \frac{4}{60}$$
$$x = 0.066 \text{ mg/kg/hour}$$

---

9 Correct answer — **A**

D/A

$$\frac{0.066 \text{ mg/kg}}{60 \text{ min}} \times \frac{1{,}000 \text{ mcg}}{1 \text{ mg}} = \frac{66 \text{ mcg/kg}}{60 \text{ min}} = 1.1 \text{ mcg/kg/minute}$$

R/P

Step 1: Change milligrams to micrograms.
$$1 \text{ mg} : 1{,}000 \text{ mcg} :: 0.066 \text{ mg} : x \text{ mcg}$$
$$x = 1{,}000 \times 0.066$$
$$x = 66 \text{ mcg/hour}$$

Step 2: Calculate micrograms per minute.

$$60 \text{ min} : 66 \text{ mcg} :: 1 \text{ min} : x \text{ mcg}$$
$$60x = 66$$
$$x = \frac{66}{60}$$
$$x = 1.1 \text{ mcg/kg/minute}$$

10 Correct answer — **A**

D/A

$$\frac{16 \cancel{U}}{1 \text{ hr}} \times \frac{\overset{5}{\cancel{250}} \text{ ml}}{\underset{2}{\cancel{100}} \cancel{U}} = \frac{80 \text{ ml}}{2 \text{ hr}} = 40 \text{ ml/hour}$$

R/P

Step 1: Calculate units administered in a milliliter.

$$250 \text{ ml} : 100 \text{ U} :: 1 \text{ ml} : x \text{ U}$$
$$250x = 100$$
$$x = \frac{100}{250}$$
$$x = 0.4 \text{ U}$$

Step 2: Calculate milliliters per hour.

$$0.4 \text{ U} : 1 \text{ ml/hr} :: 16 \text{ U} : x \text{ ml/hr}$$
$$0.4x = 16$$
$$x = \frac{16}{0.4}$$
$$x = 40 \text{ ml/hour}$$

11 Correct answer — **B**

D/A

$$\frac{\overset{4}{\cancel{40}} \text{ ml}}{\underset{6}{70 \text{ kg}/\cancel{60} \text{ min}}} \times \frac{\overset{2}{\cancel{100}} \text{ U}}{\underset{5}{\cancel{250}} \cancel{ml}} =$$

$$\frac{8 \text{ U}}{2,100 \text{ kg/min}} = 0.0038 \text{ or } 0.004 \text{ U/kg/minute}$$

R/P

Step 1: Calculate units administered in a minute.

$$60 \text{ min} : 16 \text{ U} :: 1 \text{ min} : x \text{ U}$$
$$60x = 16$$
$$x = \frac{16}{60}$$
$$x = 0.266 \text{ U}$$

Step 2: Calculate units per kilogram per minute.

$$70 \text{ kg} : 0.226 \text{ U} :: 1 \text{ kg} : x \text{ U}$$
$$70x = 0.266$$
$$x = \frac{0.266}{70}$$
$$x = 0.0038 \text{ or } 0.004 \text{ U/kg/minute}$$

12 Correct answer — **D**

D/A

$$\frac{\overset{2}{\cancel{100}} \text{ U}}{\underset{5}{\cancel{250}} \text{ ml}} = \frac{2}{5} \text{ or } 2{:}5$$

R/P

$$100 \text{ U} : 250 \text{ ml} :: 1 \text{ U} : x \text{ ml}$$
$$100x = 250$$
$$x = \frac{250}{100}$$
$$x = 2.5 \text{ ml}$$

Therefore, the concentration is 1:2.5 or 2:5

13 Correct answer — **B**

D/A

$$2{:}5 = {}^2\!/_5 = 0.4 \text{ or } 0.40 = 40\%$$

R/P

$$250 \text{ ml} : 100 \text{ U} :: 100 \text{ ml} : x \text{ U}$$
$$250x = 10{,}000$$
$$x = \frac{10{,}000}{250}$$
$$x = 40 \text{ or } 40\%$$

14 Correct answer — **D**

D/A

$$24 \, \cancel{\text{hr}} \times \frac{60 \, \cancel{\text{min}}}{1 \, \cancel{\text{hr}}} \times \frac{166.6 \, \cancel{\text{mcg}}}{1 \, \cancel{\text{min}}} \times \frac{1 \, \cancel{\text{mg}}}{1{,}000 \, \cancel{\text{mcg}}} \times \frac{\overset{1}{\cancel{250}} \text{ ml}}{\underset{1}{\cancel{250}} \, \cancel{\text{mg}}} =$$

$$\frac{239{,}904 \text{ ml}}{1{,}000} = 239.9 \text{ or } 240 \text{ ml}$$

R/P

Step 1: Change micrograms to milligrams.

$$1{,}000 \text{ mcg} : 1 \text{ mg} :: 166.6 \text{ mcg} : x \text{ mg}$$
$$1{,}000x = 166.6$$
$$x = \frac{166.6}{1{,}000}$$
$$x = 0.1666 \text{ mg}$$

Step 2: Calculate milliliters per minute.

Because the order reads 250 mg in 250 ml, there are 0.1666 ml/minute

Step 3: Calculate milliliters per hour.

$$1 \text{ min} : 0.1666 \text{ ml} :: 60 \text{ min} : x \text{ ml}$$
$$x = 0.1666 \times 60$$
$$x = 9.996 \text{ ml/hour}$$

Step 4: Calculate milliliters administered in 24 hours.

$$1 \text{ hr} : 9.996 \text{ ml} :: 24 \text{ hr} : x \text{ ml}$$
$$x = 9.996 \times 24$$
$$x = 239.9 \text{ or } 240 \text{ ml}$$

15 Correct answer—**B**

D/A

$$70 \text{ kg} \times \frac{3.6 \text{ mcg}}{\text{kg/min}} \times \frac{1 \text{ mg}}{\underset{100}{1{,}000 \text{ mcg}}} \times \frac{\overset{1}{500 \text{ ml}}}{\underset{1}{500 \text{ mg}}} \times \frac{\overset{6}{60 \text{ min}}}{1 \text{ hr}} =$$

$$\frac{1{,}512 \text{ ml}}{100 \text{ hr}} = 15.12 \text{ or } 15 \text{ ml/hour}$$

R/P

Step 1: Calculate micrograms administered in a minute.

$$1 \text{ kg} : 3.6 \text{ mcg/min} :: 70 \text{ kg} : x \text{ mcg/minute}$$
$$x = 3.6 \times 70$$
$$x = 252 \text{ mcg}$$

Step 2: Change micrograms to milligrams.

$$1{,}000 \text{ mcg} : 1 \text{ mg} :: 252 \text{ mcg} : x \text{ mg}$$
$$1{,}000x = 252$$
$$x = \frac{252}{1{,}000}$$
$$x = 0.252 \text{ mg}$$

Step 3: Calculate milligrams per hour.
$$1 \text{ min} : 0.252 \text{ mg} :: 60 \text{ min} : x \text{ mg}$$
$$x = 0.252 \times 60$$
$$x = 15.12 \text{ or } 15 \text{ mg/hour}$$

Because 500 mg of dopamine are in 500 ml of solution, the ratio of milliliters is 1:1. Therefore, 15 mg/hr = 15 ml/hour.

16 Correct answer — C

D/A

Flow rate for cefazolin (Ancef):

$$\frac{100 \text{ ml}}{60 \text{ min}} \times \frac{60 \text{ mcgtt}}{1 \text{ ml}} = 100 \text{ mcgtt/minute}$$

Flow rate for metronidazole (Flagyl):

$$\frac{50 \text{ ml}}{30 \text{ min}} \times \frac{60 \text{ mcgtt}}{1 \text{ ml}} = 100 \text{ mcgtt/minute}$$

Flow rate for heparin:

$$\frac{500 \text{ U}}{60 \text{ min}} \times \frac{250 \text{ ml}}{12,500 \text{ U}} \times \frac{60 \text{ mcgtt}}{1 \text{ ml}} = \frac{250 \text{ mcgtt}}{25 \text{ min}} = 10 \text{ mcgtt/minute}$$

R/P

To determine the flow rate for cefazolin:

Step 1: Calculate microdrops per hour.
$$1 \text{ ml} : 60 \text{ mcgtt/hr} :: 100 \text{ ml} : x \text{ mcgtt/hr}$$
$$x = 60 \times 100$$
$$x = 6,000 \text{ mcgtt/hour}$$

Step 2: Calculate microdrops per minute.
$$60 \text{ min} : 6,000 \text{ mcgtt} :: 1 \text{ min} : x \text{ mcgtt}$$
$$60x = 6,000$$
$$x = \frac{6,000}{60}$$
$$x = 100 \text{ mcgtt/minute}$$

To determine the flow rate for metronidazole:

Step 1: Calculate microdrops administered in 30 minutes.
$$1 \text{ ml} : 60 \text{ mcgtt} :: 50 \text{ ml} : x \text{ mcgtt}$$
$$x = 60 \times 50$$
$$x = 3,000 \text{ mcgtt}$$

Step 2: Calculate microdrops per minute.
$$30 \text{ min} : 3,000 \text{ mcgtt} :: 1 \text{ min} : x \text{ mcgtt}$$
$$30x = 3,000$$
$$x = \frac{3,000}{30}$$
$$x = 100 \text{ mcgtt/minute}$$

To determine the flow rate for heparin:

Step 1: Calculate required microdrops.
$$1 \text{ ml} : 60 \text{ mcgtt} :: 250 \text{ ml} : x \text{ mcgtt}$$
$$x = 60 \times 250$$
$$x = 15,000 \text{ mcgtt}$$

Step 2: Determine required minutes.
$$500 \text{ U} : 60 \text{ min} :: 12,500 \text{ U} : x \text{ min}$$
$$500x = 60 \times 12,500$$
$$x = \frac{750,000}{500}$$
$$x = 1,500 \text{ minutes}$$

Step 3: Calculate microdrops per minute.
$$1,500 \text{ min} : 15,000 \text{ mcgtt} :: 1 \text{ min} : x \text{ mcgtt}$$
$$1,500x = 15,000$$
$$x = \frac{15,000}{1,500}$$
$$x = 10 \text{ mcgtt/minute}$$

17 Correct answer — **D**

Remember: When each IVPB solution is infusing, the primary solution is not infusing.

D/A

Total volume of cefazolin in 24 hours:

$$\overset{6}{\cancel{24} \text{ hr}} \times \frac{100 \text{ ml/hr}}{\cancel{4 \text{ hr}}} = 600 \text{ ml over 6 hours IVPB}$$

Total volume of metronidazole in 24 hours:

$$\overset{4}{\cancel{24} \text{ hr}} \times \frac{50 \text{ ml/0.5 hr}}{\cancel{6 \text{ hr}}} = 200 \text{ ml over 2 hours IVPB}$$

The total IVPB volume:

$$\begin{array}{l} 600 \text{ ml cefazolin over 6 hours} \\ + \underline{\ 200 \text{ ml metronidazozle over 2 hours}} \\ 800 \text{ ml over 8 hours} \end{array}$$

Total volume of heparin in 24 hours:

$$24 \ \cancel{hr} \times \frac{\overset{1}{\cancel{500}} \ \cancel{U}}{1 \ \cancel{hr}} \times \frac{250 \ ml}{\underset{25}{\cancel{12,500}} \ \cancel{U}} =$$

$$\frac{6,000 \ ml}{25} = 240 \ ml \ daily \ via \ the \ central \ line$$

Totals:

$$\begin{array}{r} 800 \ ml \ IVPB \\ + \, 240 \ ml \ Central \\ \hline 1,040 \ ml \ Secondary \ lines \end{array}$$

8 hours committed for IVPB therapy

$$\begin{array}{rl} Order: & 2,400 \ ml \ in \ 24 \ hours \\ Secondary: - & 1,040 \ ml \ in \ 8 \ hours \\ \hline Balance: & 1,360 \ ml \ in \ 16 \ hours \ for \ the \ primary \ line \end{array}$$

$$\frac{1,360 \ \cancel{ml}}{16 \ \cancel{hr}} \times \frac{60 \ mcgtt}{1 \ \cancel{ml}} \times \frac{1 \ \cancel{hr}}{60 \ min} =$$

$$\frac{1,360 \ mcgtt}{16 \ min} = 85 \ mcgtt/minute \ for \ primary \ line$$

R/P

The total volume of cefazolin per 24 hours:

$$4 \ hr : 100 \ ml :: 24 \ hr : x \ ml$$
$$4x = 100 \times 24$$
$$x = \frac{2,400}{4}$$
$$x = 600 \ ml$$

Total time for infusion of cefazolin:

$$100 \ ml : 1 \ hr :: 600 \ ml : x \ hr$$
$$100x = 600$$
$$x = \frac{600}{100}$$
$$x = 6 \ hours \ IVPB$$

Total volume of metronidazole in 24 hours:

$$6 \ hours : 50 \ ml :: 24 \ hours : x \ ml$$
$$6x = 50 \times 24$$
$$x = \frac{1,200}{6}$$
$$x = 200 \ ml$$

Total time for infusion of metronidazole:
$$50 \text{ ml} : 0.5 \text{ hr} :: 200 \text{ ml} : x \text{ hr}$$
$$50x = 0.5 \times 200$$
$$x = \frac{100}{50}$$
$$x = 2 \text{ hours IVPB}$$

Total volume of heparin in 24 hours:

Step 1: Calculate number of units per milliliter.
$$250 \text{ ml} : 12{,}500 \text{ U} :: 1 \text{ ml} : x \text{ U}$$
$$250x = 12{,}500$$
$$x = \frac{12{,}500}{250}$$
$$x = 50 \text{ U/ml}$$

Step 2: Calculate the number of milliliters per hour.
$$50 \text{ U} : 1 \text{ ml} :: 500 \text{ U} : x \text{ ml}$$
$$50x = 500$$
$$x = \frac{500}{50}$$
$$x = 10 \text{ ml/hour}$$

Step 3: Calculate the 24-hour total.
$$1 \text{ hr} : 10 \text{ ml} :: 24 \text{ hr} : x \text{ ml}$$
$$x = 10 \times 24$$
$$x = 240 \text{ ml daily for central line}$$

$$\begin{array}{r} 800 \text{ ml IVPB} \\ + 240 \text{ ml IVPB} \\ \hline 1{,}040 \text{ ml for secondary lines} \end{array}$$

8 hours committed for IVPB therapy

$$\text{Order:} \quad \begin{array}{r} 2{,}400 \text{ ml in 24 hours restriction} \\ -1{,}040 \text{ ml in 8 hours} \\ \hline \end{array}$$

Balance: 1,360 ml in 16 hours for the primary infusion

To determine the primary infusion flow rate:

Step 1: Change milliliters to microdrops.
$$1 \text{ ml} : 60 \text{ mcgtt} :: 1{,}360 \text{ ml} : x \text{ mcgtt}$$
$$x = 60 \times 1{,}360$$
$$x = 81{,}600 \text{ mcgtt}$$

Step 2: Calculate required minutes.
$$1 \text{ hr} : 60 \text{ min} :: 16 \text{ hr} : x \text{ min}$$
$$x = 60 \times 16$$
$$x = 960 \text{ minutes}$$

Step 3: Calculate the flow rate.

$$960 \text{ min} : 81{,}600 \text{ mcgtt} :: 1 \text{ min} : x \text{ mcgtt}$$
$$960x = 81{,}600$$
$$x = \frac{81{,}600}{960}$$
$$x = 85 \text{ mcgtt/minute for primary line}$$

18 Correct answer — **A**

D/A

$$50 \text{ ml} \times \frac{\overset{1}{\cancel{50} \text{ g}}}{\underset{2}{\cancel{100} \text{ ml}}} = \frac{50 \text{ g}}{2} = 25 \text{ g}$$

R/P

$$100 \text{ ml} : 50 \text{ g} :: 50 \text{ ml} : x \text{ g}$$
$$100x = 50 \times 50$$
$$x = \frac{2{,}500}{100}$$
$$x = 25 \text{ g}$$

19 Correct answer — **B**

D/A

A 50% solution (50 ml) contains 25 g, so:

$$450 \text{ ml} + 50 \text{ ml} = 500 \text{ ml with } 25 \text{ g}$$
$$\frac{25 \text{ g}}{500 \text{ ml}} = \frac{1}{20} = 1{:}20 \ (5{:}100) \text{ or } 5\%$$

R/P

A 50% solution (50 ml) contains 25 g, so:
$$450 \text{ ml} + 50 \text{ ml} = 500 \text{ ml with } 25 \text{ g}$$
$$25 \text{ g} : 500 \text{ ml} :: 1 \text{ g} : x \text{ ml}$$
$$25x = 500$$
$$x = \frac{500}{25}$$
$$x = 20 \text{ ml} = 1{:}20 \ (5{:}100) \text{ or } 5\%$$

20 Correct answer — **D**

D/A

$$75 \text{ kg} \times \frac{10 \text{ ml}}{1 \text{ kg}} = 750 \text{ ml}$$

R/P

$$1 \text{ kg} : 10 \text{ ml} :: 75 \text{ kg} : x \text{ ml}$$
$$x = 10 \times 75$$
$$x = 750 \text{ ml}$$

21 Correct answer — **B**

D/A

$$\frac{750 \text{ ml}}{24 \text{ hr}} = 31.2 \text{ or } 31 \text{ ml/hour}$$

R/P

$$24 \text{ hr} : 750 \text{ ml} :: 1 \text{ hr} : x \text{ ml}$$
$$24x = 750$$
$$x = \frac{750}{24}$$
$$x = 31.2 \text{ or } 31 \text{ ml/hour}$$

22 Correct answer — **B**

D/A

$$\frac{31.25 \text{ ml}}{\overset{}{\underset{6}{60}} \text{ min}} \times \frac{\overset{1}{10} \text{ gtt}}{1 \text{ ml}} = \frac{31.25 \text{ gtt}}{6 \text{ min}} = 5.2 \text{ or } 5 \text{ gtt/minute}$$

R/P

Step 1: Change milliliters to drops.

$$1 \text{ ml} : 10 \text{ gtt} :: 750 \text{ ml} : x \text{ gtt}$$
$$x = 10 \times 750$$
$$x = 7,500 \text{ gtt}$$

Step 2: Calculate required minutes.

$$31.25 \text{ ml} : 60 \text{ min} :: 750 \text{ ml} : x \text{ min}$$
$$31.25x = 60 \times 750$$
$$x = \frac{45,000}{31.25}$$
$$x = 1,440 \text{ minutes}$$

Step 3: Calculate the flow rate.

$$1,440 \text{ min} : 7,500 \text{ gtt} :: 1 \text{ min} : x \text{ gtt}$$
$$1,440x = 7,500$$
$$x = \frac{7,500}{1,440}$$
$$x = 5.2 \text{ or } 5 \text{ gtt/minute}$$

23 Correct answer—**C**

D/A

Flow rates for doxapram:

Solution I:

$$\frac{5 \text{ mg}}{1 \text{ min}} \times \frac{\overset{5}{\cancel{250}} \text{ ml}}{\underset{8}{\cancel{400}} \text{ mg}} \times \frac{10 \text{ gtt}}{1 \text{ ml}} = \frac{250 \text{ gtt}}{8 \text{ min}} = 31.2 \text{ or } 31 \text{ gtt/minute}$$

Solution II:

$$\frac{3 \text{ mg}}{1 \text{ min}} \times \frac{\overset{5}{\cancel{250}} \text{ ml}}{\underset{8}{\cancel{400}} \text{ mg}} \times \frac{10 \text{ gtt}}{1 \text{ ml}} = \frac{150 \text{ gtt}}{8 \text{ min}} = 18.7 \text{ or } 19 \text{ gtt/minute}$$

Solution III:

$$\frac{1 \text{ mg}}{1 \text{ min}} \times \frac{\overset{5}{\cancel{250}} \text{ ml}}{\underset{8}{\cancel{400}} \text{ mg}} \times \frac{10 \text{ gtt}}{1 \text{ ml}} = \frac{50 \text{ gtt}}{8 \text{ min}} = 6.2 \text{ or } 6 \text{ gtt/minute}$$

R/P

Flow rates for doxapram:

Solution I:

Step 1: Change milliliters to drops.

$$1 \text{ ml} : 10 \text{ gtt} :: 250 \text{ ml} : x \text{ gtt}$$
$$x = 10 \times 250$$
$$x = 2,500 \text{ gtt}$$

Step 2: Calculate required minutes.

$$5 \text{ mg} : 1 \text{ min} :: 400 \text{ mg} : x \text{ min}$$
$$5x = 400$$
$$x = \frac{400}{5}$$
$$x = 80 \text{ minutes}$$

Step 3: Calculate the flow rate.

$$80 \text{ min} : 2,500 \text{ gtt} :: 1 \text{ min} : x \text{ gtt}$$
$$80x = 2,500$$
$$x = \frac{2,500}{80}$$
$$x = 31.2 \text{ or } 31 \text{ gtt/minute}$$

Solution II:

The number of drops are the same as above: 2,500 gtt.

Step 1: Calculate required minutes.

$$3 \text{ mg} : 1 \text{ min} :: 400 \text{ mg} : x \text{ min}$$
$$3x = 400$$
$$x = \frac{400}{3}$$
$$x = 133.5 \text{ minutes}$$

Step 2: Calculate the flow rate.

$$133.3 \text{ min} : 2,500 \text{ gtt} :: 1 \text{ min} : x \text{ gtt}$$
$$133.3x = 2,500$$
$$x = \frac{2,500}{133.3}$$
$$x = 18.7 \text{ or } 19 \text{ gtt/minute}$$

Solution III:

The number of drops are the same as above: 2,500 gtt.

Step 1: Calculate required minutes.

$$1 \text{ mg} : 1 \text{ min} :: 400 \text{ mg} : x \text{ min}$$
$$x = 400 \text{ minutes}$$

Step 2: Calculate the flow rate.

$$400 \text{ min} : 2,500 \text{ gtt} :: 1 \text{ min} : x \text{ gtt}$$
$$400x = 2,500$$
$$x = \frac{2,500}{400}$$
$$x = 6.2 \text{ or } 6 \text{ gtt/minute}$$

24 Correct answer — D

D/A
Total I.V. solution in 1 hour:

Solution I:

$$\overset{1}{\cancel{10} \text{ min}} \times \frac{31 \text{ gtt}}{1 \text{ min}} \times \frac{1 \text{ ml}}{\underset{1}{\cancel{10} \text{ gtt}}} = 31 \text{ ml in 10 minutes}$$

Solution II:

$$\overset{2}{\cancel{20} \text{ min}} \times \frac{19 \text{ gtt}}{1 \text{ min}} \times \frac{1 \text{ ml}}{\underset{1}{\cancel{10} \text{ gtt}}} = 38 \text{ ml in 20 minutes}$$

Solution III:

$$\require{cancel}\cancel{30} \overset{3}{\cancel{\text{ min}}} \times \frac{6 \text{ gtt}}{1 \text{ min}} \times \frac{1 \text{ ml}}{\underset{1}{\cancel{10} \text{ gtt}}} = 18 \text{ ml in 30 minutes}$$

$$
\begin{array}{r}
31 \text{ ml in 10 minutes} \\
38 \text{ ml in 20 minutes} \\
+18 \text{ ml in 30 minutes} \\
\hline
\end{array}
$$

Total: 87 ml in 60 minutes

R/P

Solution I:

10 gtt : 1 ml :: 31 gtt : x ml

$$10x = 31$$

$$x = \frac{31}{10}$$

$$x = 3.1 \text{ ml/min} \times 10 \text{ min} = 31 \text{ ml in 10 minutes}$$

Solution II:

10 gtt : 1 ml :: 19 gtt : x ml

$$10x = 19$$

$$x = \frac{19}{10}$$

$$x = 1.9 \text{ ml/min} \times 20 \text{ min} = 38 \text{ ml in 20 minutes}$$

Solution III:

10 gtt : 1 ml :: 6 gtt : x ml

$$10x = 6$$

$$x = \frac{6}{10}$$

$$x = 0.6 \text{ ml/min} \times 30 \text{ min} = 18 \text{ ml in 30 minutes}$$

$$
\begin{array}{r}
31 \text{ ml in 10 minutes} \\
38 \text{ ml in 20 minutes} \\
+18 \text{ ml in 30 minutes} \\
\hline
\end{array}
$$

Total: 87 ml in 60 minutes

25 Correct answer—**B**

D/A

$$\frac{\underset{1}{\overset{1}{\cancel{5} \text{ ml}}}}{\underset{12}{\cancel{40} \text{ kg}/\cancel{60} \text{ min}}} \times \frac{\overset{20}{\cancel{800} \text{ mg}}}{\underset{1}{\cancel{250} \text{ ml}}} \times \frac{\overset{4}{\cancel{1,000} \text{ mcg}}}{1 \text{ } \cancel{\text{mg}}} =$$

$$\frac{80 \text{ mcg}}{12 \text{ kg/min}} = 6.6 \text{ mcg/kg/minute for the central line}$$

R/P

Step 1: Calculate number of milligrams in 5 ml.

$$250 \text{ ml} : 800 \text{ mg} :: 5 \text{ ml} : x \text{ mg}$$
$$250x = 800 \times 5$$
$$x = \frac{4{,}000}{250}$$
$$x = 16 \text{ mg}$$

Step 2: Change milligrams to micrograms.

$$1 \text{ mg} : 1{,}000 \text{ mcg} :: 16 \text{ mg} : x \text{ mcg}$$
$$x = 1{,}000 \times 16$$
$$x = 16{,}000 \text{ mcg}$$

Step 3: Calculate required micrograms.

$$60 \text{ min} : 16{,}000 \text{ mcg} :: 1 \text{ min} : x \text{ mcg}$$
$$60x = 16{,}000$$
$$x = \frac{16{,}000}{60}$$
$$x = 266.6 \text{ mcg}$$

Step 4: Calculate micrograms per kilogram per minute.

$$40 \text{ kg} : 266.6 \text{ mcg} :: 1 \text{ kg} : x \text{ mcg}$$
$$40x = 266.6$$
$$x = \frac{266.6}{40}$$
$$x = 6.6 \text{ mcg/kg/minute for}$$
$$\text{the central line}$$

26 Correct answer — **A**

D/A

$$24 \text{ hr} \times \frac{5 \text{ ml}}{1 \text{ hr}} = 120 \text{ ml in 24 hours}$$

$$\text{IVPB} = 700 \text{ ml in 4 hours}$$

$$\begin{array}{r} 120 \text{ ml} \\ + 700 \text{ ml} \\ \hline \end{array}$$

Total: 820 ml with 4 hours for IVPB

Total I.V. fluids ordered: 1,500 ml in 24 hours
$$\begin{array}{r} - \quad 820 \text{ ml in 4 hours} \\ \hline \end{array}$$
Balance: 680 ml in 20 hours

$$\frac{680 \text{ ml}}{20 \text{ hr}} \times \frac{1 \text{ hr}}{60 \text{ min}} \times \frac{10 \text{ gtt}}{1 \text{ ml}} = \frac{68 \text{ gtt}}{12 \text{ min}} = 5.6 \text{ or } 6 \text{ gtt/minute}$$

R/P

Totals:
Central line:

$$1 \text{ hr} : 5 \text{ ml} :: 24 \text{ hr} : x \text{ ml}$$
$$x = 5 \times 24$$
$$x = 120 \text{ ml}$$

120 ml Central in 24 hours
+ 700 ml IVPB for 4 hours

Total: 820 ml for volume (4 hours for IVPB)

Total I.V. fluids ordered: 1,500 ml
− 820 ml

Balance: 680 ml in 20 hours

Step 1: Calculate required drops.
$$1 \text{ ml} : 10 \text{ gtt} :: 680 \text{ ml} : x \text{ gtt}$$
$$x = 10 \times 680$$
$$x = 6,800 \text{ gtt}$$

Step 2: Calculate required minutes.
$$1 \text{ hr} : 60 \text{ min} :: 20 \text{ hr} : x \text{ min}$$
$$x = 60 \times 20$$
$$x = 1,200 \text{ minutes}$$

Step 3: Calculate the flow rate.
$$1,200 \text{ min} : 6,800 \text{ gtt} :: 1 \text{ min} : x \text{ gtt}$$
$$1,200x = 6,800$$
$$x = \frac{6,800}{1,200}$$
$$x = 5.6 \text{ or } 6 \text{ gtt/minute for primary line}$$

27 Correct answer—**B**

D/A

$$\frac{\overset{3}{\cancel{150} \text{ mcgtt}}}{\underset{1}{\cancel{50} \text{ kg/min}}} \times \frac{1 \cancel{\text{ml}}}{60 \cancel{\text{mcgtt}}} \times \frac{\overset{2}{\cancel{500} \text{ mg}}}{\underset{1}{\cancel{250} \cancel{\text{ml}}}} =$$

$$\frac{6 \text{ mg}}{60 \text{ kg/min}} = 0.1 \text{ mg/kg/minute}$$

R/P

Step 1: Change milliliters to microdrops.
$$1 \text{ ml} : 60 \text{ mcgtt} :: 250 \text{ ml} : x \text{ mcgtt}$$
$$x = 60 \times 250$$
$$x = 15,000 \text{ mcgtt}$$

Step 2: Calculate required milligrams.

$$15{,}000 \text{ mcgtt} : 500 \text{ mg} :: 150 \text{ mcgtt} : x \text{ mg}$$
$$15{,}000x = 500 \times 150$$
$$x = \frac{75{,}000}{15{,}000}$$
$$x = 5 \text{ mg}$$

Step 3: Calculate milligrams per kilogram per minute.

$$50 \text{ kg} : 5 \text{ mg} :: 1 \text{ kg} : x \text{ mg}$$
$$50x = 5$$
$$x = \frac{5}{50}$$
$$x = 0.1 \text{ mg/kg/minute}$$

28 Correct answer — C

D/A

$$\overset{1}{\cancel{50 \text{ kg}}} \times \frac{4 \cancel{\text{mcg}}}{\cancel{\text{kg}}/\text{min}} \times \frac{1 \cancel{\text{mg}}}{\underset{20}{1{,}000 \cancel{\text{mcg}}}} \times \frac{\overset{1}{250} \cancel{\text{ml}}}{\underset{2}{500 \cancel{\text{mg}}}} \times \frac{60 \text{ mcgtt}}{1 \cancel{\text{ml}}} =$$

$$\frac{240 \text{ mcgtt}}{40 \text{ min}} = 6 \text{ mcgtt/minute}$$

R/P

Step 1: Change milligrams to micrograms.

$$1 \text{ mg} : 1{,}000 \text{ mcg} :: 0.1 \text{ mg} : x \text{ mcg}$$
$$x = 1{,}000 \times 0.1$$
$$x = 100 \text{ mcg}$$

Step 2: Calculate the flow rate.

$$100 \text{ mcg} : 150 \text{ mcgtt} :: 4 \text{ mcg} : x \text{ mcgtt}$$
$$100x = 150 \times 4$$
$$x = \frac{600}{100}$$
$$x = 6 \text{ mcgtt/minute}$$

29 Correct answer — A

D/A

$$\frac{18 \cancel{\text{gtt}}}{1 \cancel{\text{min}}} \times \frac{1 \cancel{\text{ml}}}{\underset{1}{10 \cancel{\text{gtt}}}} \times \frac{\overset{1}{50} \text{U}}{\underset{5}{250 \cancel{\text{ml}}}} \times \frac{\overset{6}{60 \cancel{\text{min}}}}{1 \text{ hr}} = \frac{108 \text{ U}}{5 \text{ hr}} = 21.6 \text{ U/hour}$$

R/P

Step 1: Calculate units per milliliter.

$$250 \text{ ml} : 50 \text{ U} :: 1 \text{ ml} : x \text{ U}$$
$$250x = 50$$
$$x = \frac{50}{250}$$
$$x = 0.2 \text{ U/ml}$$

Step 2: Calculate units per minute.

$$10 \text{ gtt} : 0.2 \text{ U} :: 18 \text{ gtt} : x \text{ U}$$
$$10x = 0.2 \times 18$$
$$x = \frac{3.6}{10}$$
$$x = 0.36 \text{ U/minute}$$

Step 3: Calculate units per hour.

$$1 \text{ min} : 0.36 \text{ U} :: 60 \text{ min} : x \text{ U}$$
$$x = 0.36 \times 60$$
$$x = 21.6 \text{ U/hour}$$

---

30 Correct answer — **D**

D/A

$$50 \cancel{U} \times \frac{1 \text{ hr}}{21.6 \cancel{U}} = \frac{50 \text{ hr}}{21.6} = 2.3 \text{ hours or 2 hours, 18 minutes}$$

R/P

$$21.6 \text{ U} : 1 \text{ hr} :: 50 \text{ U} : x \text{ hr}$$
$$21.6x = 50$$
$$x = \frac{50}{21.6}$$
$$x = 2.3 \text{ hours or 2 hours, 18 minutes}$$

---

31 Correct answer — **B**

D/A

$$\frac{50 \text{ U}}{250 \text{ ml}} = \frac{1}{5} = 1{:}5 \ (20{:}100) \text{ or } 20\%$$

R/P

$$250 \text{ ml} : 50 \text{ U} :: 100 \text{ ml} : x \text{ U}$$
$$250x = 50 \times 100$$
$$x = \frac{5{,}000}{250}$$
$$x = 20 \text{ U in 100 ml or 20\%}$$

CHAPTER 9

Comprehensive Examination

Questions

1 How many grams equal ¹⁄₁₀₀ gr?

A. ¹⁄₁₅,₀₀₀ g
B. 0.015 g
C. 0.06 g
D. 0.0007 g

2 How many centimeters equal 5½'?

A. 13.75 cm
B. 162.5 cm
C. 165 cm
D. 1,560 cm

3 38.3° C equal how many degrees Fahrenheit?

A. 99.6° F
B. 100° F
C. 100.9° F
D. 102.4° F

4 The physician orders 0.15 g of the antiulcer drug ranitidine hydrochloride (Zantac) for a patient. Available tablets contain 150 mg each. How many tablets should the nurse administer?

A. ½ tablet
B. 1 tablet
C. 1½ tablets
D. 5 tablets

5 The physician orders 0.3 ml of Lugol's solution (strong iodine solution) three times daily for a patient who is scheduled for a thyroidectomy. How many minims are in each dose?

A. 1 ℳ
B. 3 ℳ
C. 5 ℳ
D. 10 ℳ

6 A 65-kg patient is to receive 500 ml of dextrose 5% in water (D₅W) with 300 mg of dopamine (Intropin) at a rate of 3 mcg/kg/minute. The drop factor is 60 mcgtt = 1 ml. The nurse correctly calculates the flow rate to be:

A. 5 mcgtt/minute
B. 7 mcgtt/minute
C. 10 mcgtt/minute
D. 20 mcgtt/minute

7 A 10-year-old child has 80 ml of intravenous fluid left to be infused. The I.V. has a flow rate of 50 mcgtt/minute and a tubing calibration of 60 mcgtt = 1 ml. If the current time is 3 p.m., the nurse should tell the child that the infusion will be over at:

A. 3:20 p.m.
B. 4:20 p.m.
C. 4:36 p.m.
D. 4:40 p.m.

8 The pediatrician's order reads "Administer methotrexate (Mexate) 3.3 mg/m² I.M. The child's body-surface area (BSA) is 0.56 m². How many milligrams of this antineoplastic agent should be administered?

A. 0.08 mg
B. 1.8 mg
C. 2.18 mg
D. 18 mg

9 How many grams of boric acid powder, an antiseptic, are needed to prepare 2,000 ml of a 2% solution?

A. 0.004 g
B. 0.4 g
C. 4 g
D. 40 g

10 A patient must receive 150 mg of the bronchodilator oxtriphylline syrup (Choledyl) P.O. The label on the bottle reads: 50 mg = 5 ml. How many fluidounces should the nurse administer?

A. ½ f℥
B. 1½ f℥
C. 3 f℥
D. 5 f℥

11 A child is to receive 25,000 U/kg of penicillin V potassium (Pen-Vee-K) daily. Each tablet of this antibiotic contains 200,000 U (125 mg). The child weighs 66 lb. How many tablets equal the daily dose?

A. 4 tablets
B. 5 tablets
C. 7 tablets
D. 7½ tablets

12 The physician's order reads "Administer digoxin (Lanoxin) 0.125 mg I.M." How many milliliters should the nurse administer if she prepares the injection from an ampule labeled 0.5 mg in 2 ml?

A. 0.125 ml
B. 0.5 ml
C. 1 ml
D. 5 ml

13 The pediatric nurse performs a physical assessment of an infant during a well-baby checkup. The infant measures 62.5 cm. How many inches does this equal?

A. 22½"
B. 23"
C. 25"
D. 27½"

14 The label on a bottle of oral digoxin reads: 1 ml = 50 mcg. If the physician orders 0.08 mg P.O., how many milliliters of this antiarrhythmic drug should the nurse administer?

A. 1.6 ml
B. 10 ml
C. 11.2 ml
D. 24 ml

15 A drug is available in 400-mg scored tablets. If the physician orders 1.4 g of the drug, how many tablets should the nurse administer?

A. ½ tablet
B. 2 tablets
C. 3½ tablets
D. 4½ tablets

16 The physician orders the nurse to add dihydroergotamine mesylate-heparin-lidocaine (Embolex) to the 1,000 ml of D_5W a patient is receiving as parenteral therapy. If the infusion is set at a rate of 20 U/minute, how many units of this anticoagulant agent must be added to the I.V. solution to run for 24 hours?

A. 1,440 U
B. 28,800 U
C. 112,000 U
D. 288,000 U

17 If 400 ml of solution are left in the I.V. bag of a patient who is receiving 60 gtt/minute and the drop factor is 20 gtt = 1 ml, how long will the solution continue to infuse?

A. 1 hour, 2 minutes
B. 1 hour, 26 minutes
C. 2 hours, 5 minutes
D. 2 hours, 13 minutes

18 The nurse prepares to administer an order for pentobarbital (Nembutal) 0.15 g I.M. If the drug is labeled 50 mg = 1 ml, how many milliliters should she give?

A. 0.3 ml
B. 3 ml
C. 6 ml
D. 15 ml

19 How many grams of pure drug are needed to prepare 3,000 ml of a 2% neomycin-polymixin B (Neosporin) antibiotic solution?

A. 0.2 g
B. 6 g
C. 60 g
D. 150 g

20 The physician's order for a patient who is on I.V. insulin therapy reads "Add 200 U of regular insulin to 500 ml normal saline solution, and administer at 10 U/hour." How many milliliters per hour will the patient receive of this hormone solution?

A. 10 ml/hour
B. 15 ml/hour
C. 25 ml/hour
D. 35 ml/hour

21 The physician orders 500 mg of cefadroxil (Duricef) suspension P.O. The label reads "125 mg/5 ml." How many milliliters of this antibiotic should the nurse administer?

A. 4 ml
B. 5 ml
C. 9 ml
D. 20 ml

22 The physician orders 500 mg of carbenicillin disodium (Geopen) I.M. The vial contains 5 g of powder. The packet insert reads "Add 13.2 ml of sterile water to the vial. The resulting solution yields 3 ml = 1 g." How many milliliters of solution would contain the prescribed dose of this antibiotic?

A. 0.5 ml
B. 1.5 ml
C. 3 ml
D. 15 ml

23 The physician's order for a 15-kg child reads "Administer atropine sulfate 0.01 mg/kg I.M." The ampule is labeled 0.3 mg/ml. How many milliliters of this anticholinergic drug should the nurse prepare?

A. 0.5 ml
B. 1 ml
C. 1.5 ml
D. 11 ml

24 A patient is receiving an infusion at a rate of 30 mcgtt/minute. How many milliliters per hour will the patient receive if the drop factor is 60 mcgtt = 1 ml?

A. 30 ml/hour
B. 60 ml/hour
C. 120 ml/hour
D. 300 ml/hour

25 How many grams of sodium chloride are needed to prepare 2,000 ml of an isotonic (0.9%) saline solution?

A. 1 g
B. 6 g
C. 18 g
D. 36 g

26 The nurse prepares a 200-mcg dose of the antihypertensive drug clonidine (Catapres). If each tablet equals 0.1 mg, the nurse should give the patient:

A. 2 tablets
B. 3 tablets
C. 5 tablets
D. 10 tablets

27 The physician orders 1.25 mg/kg of a drug to be given I.V. in 3 hours. If the drug vial is labeled 50 mg = 10 ml and the patient weighs 65 kg, how many milliliters of the drug must be added to 100 ml of D$_5$W for the prescribed dose?

A. 1.2 ml
B. 10.25 ml
C. 16.25 ml
D. 20 ml

28 A patient is scheduled to receive 250 ml of normal saline solution I.V., to be completed in 60 minutes. The drop factor is 20 gtt = 1 ml. What will be the flow rate?

A. 8 gtt/minute
B. 64 gtt/minute
C. 83 gtt/minute
D. 143 gtt/minute

29 How many milligrams of an antacid would be included in a 10-ml container labeled 50%?

A. 50 mg
B. 150 mg
C. 500 mg
D. 5,000 mg

30 A vial labeled 2.5% contains 50 ml of a drug. What is the proportionate strength of the solution?

A. 1:2.5
B. 1:25
C. 1:40
D. 2.5:50

31 The physician orders the tissue plasminogen activator alteplase (Activase) 6 mg I.V. bolus stat. If the label on the vial reads "50 mg = 10 ml," how many milliliters should the nurse prepare?

A. 0.1 ml
B. 1.2 ml
C. 1 ml
D. 12 ml

32 The physician orders the coronary vasodilator diltiazem (Cardizem) 0.03 g P.O. for a patient. If the available tablets are labeled 30 mg each, how many tablets should be administered?

A. 1 tablet
B. 1⅓ tablets
C. 3 tablets
D. 10 tablets

33 The physician orders 10 mg/kg of a medication for a patient who weighs 110 lb. How many milligrams will the patient receive?

A. 50 mg
B. 100 mg
C. 500 mg
D. 1,100 mg

34 98.6° F equal how many degrees Celsius?

A. 36.7° C
B. 37° C
C. 38.6° C
D. 41° C

35 The physician's order reads "Administer encainide hydrochloride (Enkaid) 0.05 g P.O." If each capsule equals 50 mg, how many capsules of this oral antiarrhythmic drug should the nurse administer?

A. 1 capsule
B. 2 capsules
C. 3 capsules
D. 4 capsules

36 If a patient is to receive 40 ml of a 50% glucose solution, how many grams of glucose will he receive?

A. 20 g
B. 25 g
C. 40 g
D. 200 g

37 The nurse prepares to administer 1,000 ml of D_5W to be infused over 16 hours. If the drop factor is 20 gtt = 1 ml, what is the correct flow rate?

A. 21 gtt/minute
B. 55 gtt/minute
C. 128 gtt/minute
D. 209 gtt/minute

38 The physician orders the antitubercular drug capreomycin sulfate (Capastat) 15 mg/kg I.M. The vial is labeled 1 g = 2 ml. How many milliliters should the nurse administer if the patient weighs 70 kg?

A. 2.1 ml
B. 2.5 ml
C. 3 ml
D. 3.5 ml

39 The physician's order reads "Aztreonam (Azactam) 0.5 g q 8 to 12 hours." The vial is labeled 2 g in 15 ml. How many milliliters of this antibiotic should the nurse prepare?

A. 0.8 ml
B. 3.75 ml
C. 5 ml
D. 6 ml

40 The nurse notes that 340 ml of solution are left in a patient's I.V. bag. The solution is infusing at a rate of 30 gtt/minute, with a drop factor of 15 gtt = 1 ml. If it is currently 3 p.m., when will the infusion be completed?

A. 4:46 p.m.
B. 4:56 p.m.
C. 5:50 p.m.
D. 6:07 p.m.

41 The physician prescribes 0.08 g P.O. of the oral anticholesterol drug lovastatin (Mevacor). Each tablet contains 20 mg. How many tablets should the nurse administer?

A. 2 tablets
B. 4 tablets
C. 5 tablets
D. 6 tablets

42 The physician prescribes 0.075 mg/m² of digitoxin (Crystodigin) I.M. daily for a child with a body-surface area (BSA) of 1.1 m². How many milligrams of this antiarrhythmic drug will the child receive with each dose?

A. 0.006 mg
B. 0.06 mg
C. 0.08 mg
D. 0.2 mg

43 If a patient must receive 2.75 ml of a drug from an ampule labeled 2.5 g = 10 ml, how many milligrams will the patient receive?

A. 688 mg
B. 700 mg
C. 725 mg
D. 775 mg

44 The physician prescribes 0.5 mg P.O. of digoxin (Lanoxin) as an initial dose. Available tablets are labeled 0.25 mg each. How many tablets of this cardiac stimulant should the nurse administer?

A. ½ tablet
B. 1 tablet
C. 1½ tablets
D. 2 tablets

45 How many tablets of a drug would be needed if a patient must receive 0.004 g and each tablet contains 2 mg of the drug?

A. ½ tablet
B. 1 tablet
C. 1½ tablets
D. 2 tablets

46 The nurse prepares an infusion by adding 3 ml of a drug to 100 ml of I.V. solution. The patient is to receive 1 ml/minute. If the drop factor is 60 mcgtt = 1 ml, what is the flow rate in microdrops per minute?

A. 10 mcgtt/minute
B. 20 mcgtt/minute
C. 30 mcgtt/minute
D. 60 mcgtt/minute

47 The patient must receive 0.75 g of the antibiotic drug cefoxitin sodium (Mefoxin). The vial of powder is labeled 2 g. The directions call for adding 3.8 ml of sterile water to yield a solution of 1 ml = 500 mg. How many milliliters will contain the prescribed dose?

A. 0.05 ml
B. 0.2 ml
C. 0.5 ml
D. 1.5 ml

48 A 70-kg patient is scheduled to receive 0.5 mcg/kg/minute of nitroprusside sodium (Nipride), an antihypertensive drug. What would the flow rate be in microdrops per minute if the nurse adds 50 mg of nitroprusside sodium to 500 ml of D_5W?

A. 6 mcgtt/minute
B. 10 mcgtt/minute
C. 21 mcgtt/minute
D. 30 mcgtt/minute

49 The physician's order reads "Add 300 mg of clindamycin (Cleocin) to 50 ml of D_5W, and infuse at a rate of 10 mg/minute." If the drug is labeled 150 mg/ml, what is the adjusted flow rate in microdrops per minute?

A. 10 mcgtt/minute
B. 18 mcgtt/minute
C. 20 mcgtt/minute
D. 104 mcgtt/minute

50 A 42-lb child is to receive 5 mg/kg of the antitubercular drug isoniazid (Laniazid). Each tablet equals 50 mg. How many tablets are needed?

A. 1 tablet
B. 2 tablets
C. 3 tablets
D. 4 tablets

51 The nurse must prepare 200 U of insulin for an S.C. injection from a vial of concentrated insulin injection labeled 500 U/ml. How many milliliters should she prepare?

A. 0.4 ml
B. 2 ml
C. 5 ml
D. 6 ml

52 The physician orders an infusion of 50 ml of fat emulsion (Intralipid 10%) at a rate of 1 ml/minute. How long will it take this I.V. solution to infuse?

A. 7½ minutes
B. 10 minutes
C. 25 minutes
D. 50 minutes

53 If the physician prescribes 0.2 g of zidovudine (Retrovir) P.O. and each capsule contains 100 mg, how many capsules should the nurse give the patient?

A. 1 capsule
B. 2 capsules
C. 3 capsules
D. 5 capsules

54 A patient is to receive 375 mg of ascorbic acid (vitamin C) t.i.d. Scored tablets of 250 mg each are available. How many tablets should the nurse give for each dose?

A. ½ tablet
B. 1½ tablets
C. 2 tablets
D. 2½ tablets

55 What is the difference, in percent, between a 1:4 solution and a 10% solution?

A. 5%
B. 10%
C. 15%
D. No difference

56 The physician prescribes 200 mg of zidovudine to be given P.O. every 4 hours. Each capsule contains 100 mg. How many capsules are required for 24 hours?

A. 6 capsules
B. 8 capsules
C. 12 capsules
D. 16 capsules

57 A patient is to receive 60 mg of the antipsychotic drug loxapine succinate (Loxitane) P.O. If the drug is available in an oral concentration of 25 mg/ml, how many milliliters should the nurse administer?

A. 0.5 ml
B. 1 ml
C. 2.4 ml
D. 3 ml

58 The nurse is instructed to add 31.6 ml to a 20 million-U vial of the antibiotic penicillin G sodium so that 1 ml = 500,000 U. How many milliliters would equal 1.2 million U of this drug?

A. 2 ml
B. 2.4 ml
C. 5 ml
D. 24 ml

59 The nurse must add 100 mg of a drug (10 mg = 1 ml) to 500 ml D_5W and infuse at a rate of 500 mcg/minute. What will be the flow rate, in microdrops per minute, of this 510-ml solution if the drop factor is 60 mcgtt = 1 ml?

A. 15 mcgtt/minute
B. 53 mcgtt/minute
C. 84 mcgtt/minute
D. 153 mcgtt/minute

60 The physician prescribes 25 mg/kg of oxtriphylline (Choledyl) for a 40-kg patient. How many milliliters should the nurse prepare if the bottle is labeled 5 ml = 50 mg?

A. 25 ml
B. 50 ml
C. 100 ml
D. 264 ml

61 A patient with uncomplicated gonorrhea is scheduled to receive 1 g of an antibiotic by I.M. injection. How many milliliters should the nurse prepare if the vial reads 270 mg = 1 ml?

A. 0.3 ml
B. 1 ml
C. 3.7 ml
D. 5 ml

62 The physician orders two vials of 25% serum albumin I.V. for a patient. Each vial contains 50 ml. How many total grams are contained in two vials of this protein?

A. 25 g
B. 50 g
C. 250 g
D. 400 g

63 The nurse adds 20 ml of diluent to a vial containing 1 g of a drug. How many minims equal 25 mg of the drug?

A. 7.5 ℳ
B. 9 ℳ
C. 10 ℳ
D. 16 ℳ

64 The physician writes an order for 400,000 U of aqueous penicillin G by I.M. injection. The nurse prepares the injection by adding 23 ml of diluent to a 5 million-U vial, so that 1 ml = 200,000 U. How many milliliters equals 400,000 U?

A. 0.6 ml
B. 1 ml
C. 1.2 ml
D. 2 ml

65 The physician orders 75 mg of captopril (Capoten) for a patient. If each tablet of this antihypertensive drug contains 37.5 mg, the nurse should administer:

A. 1 tablet
B. 2 tablets
C. 4 tablets
D. 5 tablets

66 The physician's order reads "Metronidazole (Flagyl), 0.5 g I.V. in 100 ml D_5W, to infuse over 30 minutes." What will be the flow rate if the drop factor is 60 mcgtt = 1 ml?

A. 200 mcgtt/minute
B. 215 mcgtt/minute
C. 230 mcgtt/minute
D. 250 mcgtt/minute

67 The physician orders 10 mg/kg of an antibiotic for a patient weighing 70 kg. The vial label reads 1 ml = 400 mg. How many milliliters should the nurse prepare?

A. 0.2 ml
B. 1.3 ml
C. 1.5 ml
D. 1.75 ml

68 The physician orders 20 U of NPH insulin to be administered S.C. The label reads 1 ml = 100 U. How many milliliters of this hormone should the nurse administer to the patient?

A. 0.1 ml
B. 0.2 ml
C. 1 ml
D. 2.2 ml

69 The physician's order reads "Cimetidine (Tagamet), 300 mg in 100 ml D_5W, given by intravenous piggyback in 30 minutes." If the drop factor is 20 gtt = 1 ml, what will be the flow rate for this antiulcer medication?

A. 20 gtt/minute
B. 66 gtt/minute
C. 67 gtt/minute
D. 72 gtt/minute

70 The physician prescribes 0.25 g of ampicillin sodium (Omnipen-N) I.M. The label on the vial reads "Add 20.4 ml of sterile water to the vial, resulting in 1 ml = 500 mg." How many milliliters should the nurse administer?

A. 0.4 ml
B. 0.5 ml
C. 1 ml
D. 2 ml

71 The physician orders 0.3 mg/kg of a specific drug for a 66-kg patient. How many milliliters contain the prescribed dose if the vial is labeled 1 ml = 10 mg?

A. 0.3 ml
B. 1.8 ml
C. 2 ml
D. 2.8 ml

72 The physician has ordered 0.2 g of phenylbutazone (Butazolidin) P.O. for its anti-inflammatory properties. The only available form of this drug is scored tablets labeled 100 mg each. How many tablets should the nurse administer?

A. 1 tablet
B. 2 tablets
C. 3½ tablets
D. 10 tablets

73 The chart for a patient on the medical-surgical unit states that the patient is to receive 15 g of a drug in oral suspension form. If each teaspoon contains approximately 3.75 g of the drug, how many teaspoons should the nurse administer?

A. 1 tsp
B. 1½ tsp
C. 2 tsp
D. 4 tsp

74 A patient who is receiving I.V. therapy postoperatively has 625 ml left in the solution bag. The flow rate is listed as 100 mcgtt/minute, and the drop factor is 60 mcgtt = 1 ml. How much longer will the infusion last?

A. 1 hour, 15 minutes
B. 3 hours, 35 minutes
C. 4 hours, 20 minutes
D. 6 hours, 15 minutes

75 The nurse adds 1 gr of morphine sulfate to 1,000 ml of D_5W for infusion of a patient who is to receive 1 mg of this narcotic solution every 10 minutes. What is the flow rate in microdrops if the drop factor is 60 mcgtt = 1 ml?

A. 100 mcgtt/minute
B. 110 mcgtt/minute
C. 115 mcgtt/minute
D. 120 mcgtt/minute

76 The physician orders 5 mg/m^2 of the antiemetic dronabinol (Marinol) P.O. for a child with a BSA of 0.52 m^2. How many milligrams will the child receive?

A. 2 mg
B. 2.6 mg
C. 3.3 mg
D. 26 mg

77 The nurse's notes indicate that a patient is to receive 22 mg of a topical ointment applied daily. The pharmacy sends up a tube of ointment labeled 2.5 cm = 15 mg. How many inches of ointment should the nurse apply for each dose?

A. ½"
B. 1"
C. 1½"
D. 3"

78 The physician's order reads "Cefoxitin sodium (Mefoxin) 2 g I.V. in 150 ml D_5W." What is the flow rate in microdrops per minute if the infusion time is 90 minutes and the drop factor is 60 mcgtt = 1 ml?

A. 90 mcgtt/minute
B. 100 mcgtt/minute
C. 110 mcgtt/minute
D. 120 mcgtt/minute

79 The physician's order reads "Administer 1,000 ml of normal saline solution with 250 U of regular insulin at a rate of 13 U/hour." What is the flow rate in microdrops per minute?

A. 26 mcgtt/minute
B. 30 mcgtt/minute
C. 52 mcgtt/minute
D. 65 mcgtt/minute

80 A child is to receive 0.25 ml/kg of a drug that is labeled 2 mg/5 ml. How many milliliters should the nurse administer if the child weighs 20 kg?

A. 0.5 ml
B. 1 ml
C. 4.5 ml
D. 5 ml

81 A patient is receiving 100 ml/hour of the intravascular volume expander D_5W. If the drop factor is 15 gtt = 1 ml, what is the flow rate?

A. 25 gtt/minute
B. 35 gtt/minute
C. 50 gtt/minute
D. 60 gtt/minute

82 A child with a BSA of 0.7 m² is on maintenance antineoplastic therapy with 75 mg/m² of procarbazine (Matulane) daily. How many milligrams are in each daily dose?

A. 39 mg
B. 52.5 mg
C. 63.8 mg
D. 72 mg

83 The physician prescribes secobarbital (Seconal) 2½ gr by rectal suppository for a patient requiring sedation. If the only suppositories available on the unit are labeled 100 mg each, how many should the nurse administer?

A. 1 suppository
B. 1½ suppositories
C. 2 suppositories
D. None; the nurse should ask the pharmacy to send up correct strength

84 The physician prescribes 2 g of the antiseizure drug magnesium sulfate. How many milliliters should the nurse administer if the vial reads "Magnesium sulfate 50% in 10 ml"?

A. 4 ml
B. 5 ml
C. 5.6 ml
D. 10 ml

85 A vial of medication is labeled "50% solution." How many milliliters would be needed to administer 500 mg of medication?

A. 0.1 ml
B. 0.5 ml
C. 0.75 ml
D. 1 ml

86 The physician orders a continuous infusion of heparin for a patient weighing 52.3 kg. The order reads "Add 20,000 U of heparin to 1,000 ml normal saline solution, and infuse 0.3 U/kg/minute." The tubing is labeled as 20 gtt = 1 ml. What will be the flow rate of this anticoagulant solution?

A. 16 gtt/minute
B. 19 gtt/minute
C. 22 gtt/minute
D. 45 gtt/minute

87 The nurse adds 25 mcg of desmopressin (DDAVP) to 50 ml of normal saline solution for an infusion to be run at 0.01 mcg/kg/minute. If the patient weighs 75 kg and the drop factor is 60 mcgtt = 1 ml, what is the flow rate?

A. 39 mcgtt/minute
B. 67 mcgtt/minute
C. 90 mcgtt/minute
D. 98 mcgtt/minute

88 The order calls for 1 liter of D_5W with 500 mg of hydrocortisone (Solu-Cortef) to infuse at a rate of 0.02 mg/kg/minute. The patient weighs 66 kg, and the drop factor is 20 gtt = 1 ml. What is the correct flow rate for this glucocorticoid solution?

A. 20 gtt/minute
B. 24 gtt/minute
C. 49 gtt/minute
D. 53 gtt/minute

89 The physician orders an infusion of 150 mg of doxycycline (Vibramycin) added to 1,000 ml of D_5W for a patient weighing 40.9 kg. If the order calls for the antibiotic to run at a rate of 0.015 mg/kg/minute and the drop factor is 15 gtt = 1 ml, what is the flow rate?

A. 61 gtt/minute
B. 72 gtt/minute
C. 89 gtt/minute
D. 100 gtt/minute

90 A patient weighing 54.5 kg is scheduled to receive gentamicin (Garamycin) by I.V. drip. The nurse prepares the infusion, which is to run at 0.05 mg/kg/minute, by adding 150 mg of the drug to 200 ml of D_5W. What is the flow rate if the drop factor is 10 gtt = 1 ml?

A. 36 gtt/minute
B. 40 gtt/minute
C. 45 gtt/minute
D. 50 gtt/minute

91 A 195-lb male patient is to receive 50 mg of nitroprusside sodium (Nipride), which has been added to 1,000 ml D₅W, at a rate of 0.5 mcg/kg/minute. If the drop factor is 20 gtt = 1 ml, the nurse should adjust the flow rate for:

A. 4 gtt/minute
B. 5 gtt/minute
C. 10 gtt/minute
D. 18 gtt/minute

92 A loading dose of the bronchodilator aminophylline (Phyllocontin) is ordered for a patient weighing 116 lb. The nurse prepares the infusion by adding 300 mg of the drug to 100 ml of normal saline solution. The infusion is to run at a rate of 5.6 mg/kg over 30 minutes. If the tubing has a drop factor of 10 gtt = 1 ml, what is the adjusted flow rate?

A. 11 gtt/minute
B. 33 gtt/minute
C. 40 gtt/minute
D. 67 gtt/minute

93 An I.V. infusion of 5,000 U of heparin in 500 ml of D₅W is started for a patient weighing 154 lb. The anticoagulant solution is to infuse at a rate of 50 U/kg/hour. What is the adjusted flow rate for a drop factor of 10 gtt = 1 ml?

A. 25 gtt/minute
B. 58 gtt/minute
C. 81 gtt/minute
D. 88 gtt/minute

94 The physician orders an infusion of isoproterenol (Isuprel) for a 142-lb male patient to be infused at the rate of 0.03 mcg/kg/minute. To prepare the solution, the nurse adds 2 mg of the drug to 500 ml of D₅W. If the drop rate is 60 mcgtt = 1 ml, what is the adjusted flow rate in microdrops per minute?

A. 29 mcgtt/minute
B. 33 mcgtt/minute
C. 50 mcgtt/minute
D. 61 mcgtt/minute

95 The physician orders 0.5 g of lidocaine (Xylocaine), which is added to 1,000 ml of D_5W and infused at a rate of 0.004 mg/kg/minute, for a 125-lb patient because of the drug's antiarrhythmic action. If the drop factor is labeled as 20 gtt = 1 ml, what is the adjusted flow rate?

A. 9 gtt/minute
B. 18 gtt/minute
C. 30 gtt/minute
D. 48 gtt/minute

96 A 64-lb child is to receive the antibiotic oxacillin (Prostaphlin) I.V. by microdrop infusion at a rate of 0.3 mg/kg/30 minutes. The nurse adds 60 mg of the drug to 120 ml of 0.9% saline solution. If the drop factor is 60 mcgtt = 1 ml, the nurse should regulate the flow rate to:

A. 10 mcgtt/minute
B. 35 mcgtt/minute
C. 47 mcgtt/minute
D. 90 mcgtt/minute

97 The nurse adds 5 mg phentolamine (Regitine) to 500 ml of D_5W to be infused at a rate of 0.8 mcg/kg/minute. If the patient weighs 110 lb, and the drop factor is labeled as 10 gtt = 1 ml, what is the flow rate?

A. 20 gtt/minute
B. 40 gtt/minute
C. 44 gtt/minute
D. 105 gtt/minute

98 The physician orders dobutamine (Dobutrex), an inotropic agent, for a 138-lb patient. The order reads "Infuse 1,000 ml of D_5W with 500 mg of dobutamine at 6.5 mcg/kg/minute." The tubing has a drop factor of 60 mcgtt = 1 ml. What is the adjusted flow rate?

A. 5 mcgtt/minute
B. 10 mcgtt/minute
C. 49 mcgtt/minute
D. 83 mcgtt/minute

SITUATION

The physician prescribes dopamine hydrochloride (Intropin) to help increase the renal perfusion of a patient weighing 72 kg. The nurse adds 400 mg (5 ml) of dopamine to 500 ml D₅W, for a total infusion volume of 505 ml.

Questions 99 and 100 refer to this situation.

99 If the solution is to infuse at a rate of 3 mcg/kg/minute, what is the rate in milliliters per hour?

A. 16.3 ml/hour
B. 32.6 ml/hour
C. 72 ml/hour
D. 82 ml/hour

100 The physician decreases the infusion rate to 0.002 mg/kg/minute. How many milliliters per hour will be infusing?

A. 10.9 ml/hour
B. 12.1 ml/hour
C. 14 ml/hour
D. 31.5 ml/hour

Answer sheet

	A B C D		A B C D		A B C D		A B C D
1	○ ○ ○ ○	**31**	○ ○ ○ ○	**61**	○ ○ ○ ○	**91**	○ ○ ○ ○
2	○ ○ ○ ○	**32**	○ ○ ○ ○	**62**	○ ○ ○ ○	**92**	○ ○ ○ ○
3	○ ○ ○ ○	**33**	○ ○ ○ ○	**63**	○ ○ ○ ○	**93**	○ ○ ○ ○
4	○ ○ ○ ○	**34**	○ ○ ○ ○	**64**	○ ○ ○ ○	**94**	○ ○ ○ ○
5	○ ○ ○ ○	**35**	○ ○ ○ ○	**65**	○ ○ ○ ○	**95**	○ ○ ○ ○
6	○ ○ ○ ○	**36**	○ ○ ○ ○	**66**	○ ○ ○ ○	**96**	○ ○ ○ ○
7	○ ○ ○ ○	**37**	○ ○ ○ ○	**67**	○ ○ ○ ○	**97**	○ ○ ○ ○
8	○ ○ ○ ○	**38**	○ ○ ○ ○	**68**	○ ○ ○ ○	**98**	○ ○ ○ ○
9	○ ○ ○ ○	**39**	○ ○ ○ ○	**69**	○ ○ ○ ○	**99**	○ ○ ○ ○
10	○ ○ ○ ○	**40**	○ ○ ○ ○	**70**	○ ○ ○ ○	**100**	○ ○ ○ ○
11	○ ○ ○ ○	**41**	○ ○ ○ ○	**71**	○ ○ ○ ○		
12	○ ○ ○ ○	**42**	○ ○ ○ ○	**72**	○ ○ ○ ○		
13	○ ○ ○ ○	**43**	○ ○ ○ ○	**73**	○ ○ ○ ○		
14	○ ○ ○ ○	**44**	○ ○ ○ ○	**74**	○ ○ ○ ○		
15	○ ○ ○ ○	**45**	○ ○ ○ ○	**75**	○ ○ ○ ○		
16	○ ○ ○ ○	**46**	○ ○ ○ ○	**76**	○ ○ ○ ○		
17	○ ○ ○ ○	**47**	○ ○ ○ ○	**77**	○ ○ ○ ○		
18	○ ○ ○ ○	**48**	○ ○ ○ ○	**78**	○ ○ ○ ○		
19	○ ○ ○ ○	**49**	○ ○ ○ ○	**79**	○ ○ ○ ○		
20	○ ○ ○ ○	**50**	○ ○ ○ ○	**80**	○ ○ ○ ○		
21	○ ○ ○ ○	**51**	○ ○ ○ ○	**81**	○ ○ ○ ○		
22	○ ○ ○ ○	**52**	○ ○ ○ ○	**82**	○ ○ ○ ○		
23	○ ○ ○ ○	**53**	○ ○ ○ ○	**83**	○ ○ ○ ○		
24	○ ○ ○ ○	**54**	○ ○ ○ ○	**84**	○ ○ ○ ○		
25	○ ○ ○ ○	**55**	○ ○ ○ ○	**85**	○ ○ ○ ○		
26	○ ○ ○ ○	**56**	○ ○ ○ ○	**86**	○ ○ ○ ○		
27	○ ○ ○ ○	**57**	○ ○ ○ ○	**87**	○ ○ ○ ○		
28	○ ○ ○ ○	**58**	○ ○ ○ ○	**88**	○ ○ ○ ○		
29	○ ○ ○ ○	**59**	○ ○ ○ ○	**89**	○ ○ ○ ○		
30	○ ○ ○ ○	**60**	○ ○ ○ ○	**90**	○ ○ ○ ○		

Answers

1 Correct answer — **B**

D/A

$$\frac{1 \text{ gr}}{100} \times \frac{1 \text{ g}}{15 \text{ gr}} = \frac{1 \text{ g}}{1,500} = 0.00066 \text{ or } 0.0007 \text{ g}$$

R/P

$$15 \text{ gr} : 1 \text{ g} :: \frac{1}{100} \text{ gr} : x \text{ g}$$
$$15x = \frac{1}{100}$$
$$x = \frac{.01}{15}$$
$$x = 0.00066 \text{ or } 0.0007 \text{ g}$$

2 Correct answer — **C**

D/A

$$5.5' \times \frac{12''}{1'} \times \frac{2.5 \text{ cm}}{1''} = 165 \text{ cm}$$

R/P

Step 1: Change feet to inches.
$$1' : 12'' :: 5.5' : x ''$$
$$x = 12 \times 5.5$$
$$x = 66''$$

Step 2: Change inches to centimeters.
$$1'' : 2.5 \text{ cm} :: 66'' : x \text{ cm}$$
$$x = 2.5 \times 66$$
$$x = 165 \text{ cm}$$

3 Correct answer — **C**
Remember: This is the standard formula.

$$(°C \times 1.8) + 32 = °F$$
$$(38.3° \times 1.8) + 32° = 100.9° \text{ F}$$

4 Correct answer — **B**

D/A

$$0.15 \text{ g} \times \frac{1,000 \text{ mg}}{1 \text{ g}} \times \frac{1 \text{ tab}}{150 \text{ mg}} = \frac{150 \text{ tab}}{150} = 1 \text{ tablet}$$

R/P

$$1 \text{ g} : 1,000 \text{ mg} :: 0.15 \text{ g} : x \text{ mg}$$
$$x = 1,000 \times 0.15$$
$$x = 150 \text{ mg}$$

Because each tablet equals 150 mg, administer 1 tablet.

5 Correct answer — C

D/A

$$0.3 \text{ ml} \times \frac{15 \text{ m}}{1 \text{ ml}} = 4.5 \text{ or } 5 \text{ m}$$

R/P

$$1 \text{ ml} : 15 \text{ m} :: 0.3 \text{ ml} : x \text{ m}$$
$$x = 15 \times 0.3$$
$$x = 4.5 \text{ or } 5 \text{ m}$$

6 Correct answer — D

D/A

$$65 \text{ kg} \times \frac{3 \text{ mcg}}{\text{kg/min}} \times \frac{1 \text{ mg}}{1{,}000 \text{ mcg}} \times \frac{\overset{1}{500} \text{ ml}}{\underset{5}{300} \text{ mg}} \times \frac{\overset{1}{60} \text{ mcgtt}}{1 \text{ ml}} =$$

(with cancellations: 2 under 1,000 mcg; 5 under 300 mg)

$$\frac{195 \text{ mcgtt}}{10 \text{ min}} = 19.5 \text{ or } 20 \text{ mcgtt/minute}$$

R/P

Step 1: Change milliliters to microdrops.
$$1 \text{ ml} : 60 \text{ mcgtt} :: 500 \text{ ml} : x \text{ mcgtt}$$
$$x = 60 \times 500$$
$$x = 30{,}000 \text{ mcgtt}$$

Step 2: Calculate micrograms per minute.
$$1 \text{ kg} : 3 \text{ mcg/min} :: 65 \text{ kg} : x \text{ mcg/min}$$
$$x = 3 \times 65$$
$$x = 195 \text{ mcg/minute}$$

Step 3: Change micrograms to milligrams.
$$1{,}000 \text{ mcg} : 1 \text{ mg} :: 195 \text{ mcg} : x \text{ mg}$$
$$1{,}000x = 195$$
$$x = \frac{195}{1{,}000}$$
$$x = 0.195 \text{ mg/minute}$$

Step 4: Calculate required minutes.
$$0.195 \text{ mg} : 1 \text{ min} :: 300 \text{ mg} : x \text{ min}$$
$$0.195x = 300$$
$$x = \frac{300}{0.195}$$
$$x = 1{,}538.4 \text{ minutes}$$

Step 5: Calculate the flow rate.

$$1{,}538.4 \text{ min} : 30{,}000 \text{ mcgtt} :: 1 \text{ min} : x \text{ mcgtt}$$
$$1{,}538.4x = 30{,}000$$
$$x = \frac{30{,}000}{1{,}538.4}$$
$$x = 19.5 \text{ or } 20 \text{ mcgtt/minute}$$

7 Correct answer — C

D/A

$$80 \text{ ml} \times \frac{\overset{6}{\cancel{60}} \text{ mcgtt}}{1 \text{ ml}} \times \frac{1 \text{ min}}{\underset{5}{\cancel{50}} \text{ mcgtt}} = \frac{480 \text{ min}}{5} = 96 \text{ minutes}$$

The I.V. will end at 4:36 p.m.

R/P

Step 1: Change milliliters to microdrops.

$$1 \text{ ml} : 60 \text{ mcgtt} :: 80 \text{ ml} : x \text{ mcgtt}$$
$$x = 60 \times 80$$
$$x = 4{,}800 \text{ mcgtt}$$

Step 2: Calculate required minutes.

$$50 \text{ mcgtt} : 1 \text{ min} :: 4{,}800 \text{ mcgtt} : x \text{ min}$$
$$50x = 4{,}800$$
$$x = \frac{4{,}800}{50}$$
$$x = 96 \text{ minutes}$$

The I.V will end at 4:36 p.m.

8 Correct answer — B

D/A

$$0.56 \text{ m}^2 \times \frac{3.3 \text{ mg}}{1 \text{ m}^2} = 1.8 \text{ mg}$$

R/P

$$1 \text{ m}^2 : 3.3 \text{ mg} :: 0.56 \text{ m}^2 : x \text{ mg}$$
$$x = 3.3 \times 0.56$$
$$x = 1.8 \text{ mg}$$

9 Correct answer — D

D/A

$$2{,}000 \text{ ml} \times \frac{2 \text{ g}}{\underset{1}{\overset{20}{\cancel{100}}} \text{ ml}} = 40 \text{ g}$$

R/P

$$100 \text{ ml} : 2 \text{ g} :: 2{,}000 \text{ ml} : x \text{ g}$$
$$100x = 2 \times 2{,}000$$
$$x = \frac{4{,}000}{100}$$
$$x = 40 \text{ g}$$

10 Correct answer — **A**

D/A

$$\overset{5}{\cancel{150} \text{ mg}} \times \frac{\overset{1}{\cancel{5} \text{ ml}}}{\underset{10}{\cancel{50} \text{ mg}}} \times \frac{1 \text{ f}\text{\small ℥}}{\underset{1}{\cancel{30} \text{ ml}}} = \frac{5 \text{ f}\text{\small ℥}}{10} = \tfrac{1}{2} \text{ f}\text{\small ℥}$$

R/P

Step 1: Calculate required milliliters.
$$50 \text{ mg} : 5 \text{ ml} :: 150 \text{ mg} : x \text{ ml}$$
$$50x = 5 \times 150$$
$$x = \frac{750}{50}$$
$$x = 15 \text{ ml}$$

Step 2: Change milliliters to fluidounces.
$$30 \text{ ml} : 1 \text{ f}\text{\small ℥} :: 15 \text{ ml} : x \text{ f}\text{\small ℥}$$
$$30x = 15$$
$$x = \frac{15}{30}$$
$$x = \tfrac{1}{2} \text{ f}\text{\small ℥}$$

11 Correct answer — **A**

D/A

$$66 \; \cancel{\text{lb}} \times \frac{1 \; \cancel{\text{kg}}}{2.2 \; \cancel{\text{lb}}} \times \frac{\overset{5}{25{,}000 \; \cancel{\text{U}}}}{1 \; \cancel{\text{kg}}} \times \frac{1 \text{ tab}}{\underset{40}{200{,}000 \; \cancel{\text{U}}}} =$$

$$\frac{330 \text{ tab}}{88} = 3.75 \text{ or } 4 \text{ tablets}$$

R/P

Step 1: Change pounds to kilograms.

$$2.2 \text{ lb} : 1 \text{ kg} :: 66 \text{ lb} : x \text{ kg}$$
$$2.2x = 66$$
$$x = \frac{66}{2.2}$$
$$x = 30 \text{ kg}$$

Step 2: Calculate required units.

$$1 \text{ kg} : 25,000 \text{ U} :: 30 \text{ kg} : x \text{ U}$$
$$x = 25,000 \times 30$$
$$x = 750,000 \text{ U}$$

Step 3: Calculate required tablets.

$$200,000 \text{ U} : 1 \text{ tab} :: 750,000 \text{ U} : x \text{ tab}$$
$$200,000x = 750,000$$
$$x = \frac{750,000}{200,000}$$
$$x = 3.75 \text{ or } 4 \text{ tablets}$$

12 Correct answer — **B**

D/A

$$0.125 \text{ mg} \times \frac{2 \text{ ml}}{0.5 \text{ mg}} = \frac{0.25 \text{ ml}}{0.5} = 0.5 \text{ ml}$$

R/P

$$0.5 \text{ mg} : 2 \text{ ml} :: 0.125 \text{ mg} : x \text{ ml}$$
$$0.5x = 2 \times 0.125$$
$$x = \frac{0.25}{0.5}$$
$$x = 0.5 \text{ ml}$$

13 Correct answer — **C**

D/A

$$62.5 \text{ cm} \times \frac{1''}{2.5 \text{ cm}} = \frac{62.5''}{2.5} = 25''$$

R/P

$$2.5 \text{ cm} : 1'' :: 62.5 \text{ cm} : x''$$
$$2.5x = 62.5$$
$$x = \frac{62.5}{2.5}$$
$$x = 25''$$

14 Correct answer — **A**

D/A

$$0.08 \ \text{mg} \times \frac{\overset{100}{\cancel{1,000} \ \cancel{\text{mcg}}}}{1 \ \cancel{\text{mg}}} \times \frac{1 \ \text{ml}}{\underset{5}{\cancel{50} \ \cancel{\text{mcg}}}} = \frac{8 \ \text{ml}}{5} = 1.6 \ \text{ml}$$

R/P

Step 1: Change milligrams to micrograms.

$$1 \ \text{mg} : 1,000 \ \text{mcg} :: 0.08 \ \text{mg} : x \ \text{mcg}$$
$$x = 1,000 \times 0.08$$
$$x = 80 \ \text{mcg}$$

Step 2: Calculate required milliliters.

$$50 \ \text{mcg} : 1 \ \text{ml} :: 80 \ \text{mcg} : x \ \text{ml}$$
$$50x = 80$$
$$x = \frac{80}{50}$$
$$x = 1.6 \ \text{ml}$$

15 Correct answer — **C**

D/A

$$1.4 \ \cancel{\text{g}} \times \frac{1,000 \ \cancel{\text{mg}}}{1 \ \cancel{\text{g}}} \times \frac{1 \ \text{tab}}{400 \ \cancel{\text{mg}}} = \frac{1,400 \ \text{tab}}{400} = 3.5 \ \text{or} \ 3\frac{1}{2} \ \text{tablets}$$

R/P

Step 1: Change grams to milligrams.

$$1 \ \text{g} : 1,000 \ \text{mg} :: 1.4 \ \text{g} : x \ \text{mg}$$
$$x = 1,000 \times 1.4$$
$$x = 1,400 \ \text{mg}$$

Step 2: Calculate required tablets.

$$400 \ \text{mg} : 1 \ \text{tab} :: 1,400 \ \text{mg} : x \ \text{tab}$$
$$400x = 1,400$$
$$x = \frac{1,400}{400}$$
$$x = 3.5 \ \text{or} \ 3\frac{1}{2} \ \text{tablets}$$

16 Correct answer — **B**

D/A

$$24 \ \cancel{\text{hr}} \times \frac{60 \ \cancel{\text{min}}}{1 \ \cancel{\text{hr}}} \times \frac{20 \ \text{U}}{1 \ \cancel{\text{min}}} = 28,800 \ \text{U}$$

R/P

Step 1: Change hours to minutes.
$$1 \text{ hr} : 60 \text{ min} :: 24 \text{ hr} : x \text{ min}$$
$$x = 60 \times 24$$
$$x = 1{,}440 \text{ minutes}$$

Step 2: Calculate required units.
$$1 \text{ min} : 20 \text{ U} :: 1{,}440 \text{ min} : x \text{ U}$$
$$x = 20 \times 1{,}440$$
$$x = 28{,}800 \text{ U}$$

---

17 Correct answer — **D**

D/A

$$\frac{20}{\overset{}{400} \text{ ml}} \times \frac{\overset{1}{\cancel{20} \text{ gtt}}}{1 \text{ ml}} \times \frac{1 \text{ min}}{\underset{3}{\cancel{60} \text{ gtt}}} \times \frac{1 \text{ hr}}{\underset{3}{\cancel{60} \text{ min}}} =$$

$$\frac{20 \text{ hr}}{9} = 2.22 \text{ or 2 hours, 13 minutes}$$

R/P

Step 1: Change milliliters to drops.
$$1 \text{ ml} : 20 \text{ gtt} :: 40 \text{ ml} : x \text{ gtt}$$
$$x = 20 \times 40$$
$$x = 8{,}000 \text{ gtt}$$

Step 2: Calculate required minutes.
$$60 \text{ gtt} : 1 \text{ min} :: 8{,}000 \text{ gtt} : x \text{ min}$$
$$60x = 8{,}000$$
$$x = \frac{8{,}000}{60}$$
$$x = 133.3 \text{ minutes}$$

Step 3: Change minutes to hours.
$$60 \text{ min} : 1 \text{ hr} :: 133.3 \text{ min} : x \text{ hr}$$
$$60x = 133.3$$
$$x = \frac{133.3}{60}$$
$$x = 2.22 \text{ hours or 2 hours, 13 minutes}$$

---

18 Correct answer — **B**

D/A

$$0.15 \text{ g} \times \frac{1{,}000 \text{ mg}}{1 \text{ g}} \times \frac{1 \text{ ml}}{50 \text{ mg}} = \frac{150 \text{ ml}}{50} = 3 \text{ ml}$$

R/P

Step 1: Change grams to milligrams.

$$1 \text{ g} : 1{,}000 \text{ mg} :: 0.15 \text{ g} : x \text{ mg}$$
$$x = 1{,}000 \times 0.15$$
$$x = 150 \text{ mg}$$

Step 2: Calculate required milliliters.

$$50 \text{ mg} : 1 \text{ ml} :: 150 \text{ mg} : x \text{ ml}$$
$$50x = 150$$
$$x = \frac{150}{50}$$
$$x = 3 \text{ ml}$$

19 Correct answer—C

D/A

$$3{,}000 \text{ m\!\!/l} \times \frac{2 \text{ g}}{100 \text{ m\!\!/l}} = 60 \text{ g}$$

R/P

$$100 \text{ ml} : 2 \text{ g} :: 3{,}000 \text{ ml} : x \text{ g}$$
$$100x = 2 \times 3{,}000$$
$$x = \frac{6{,}000}{100}$$
$$x = 60 \text{ g}$$

20 Correct answer—C

D/A

$$\frac{10 \text{ \cancel{U}}}{1 \text{ hr}} \times \frac{\overset{5}{\cancel{500}} \text{ ml}}{\underset{2}{\cancel{200}} \text{ \cancel{U}}} = \frac{50 \text{ ml}}{2 \text{ hr}} = 25 \text{ ml/hour}$$

R/P

$$200 \text{ U} : 500 \text{ ml} :: 10 \text{ U} : x \text{ ml}$$
$$200x = 500 \times 10$$
$$x = \frac{5{,}000}{200}$$
$$x = 25 \text{ ml/hour}$$

21 Correct answer—**D**

D/A

$$500 \text{ mg} \times \frac{\overset{1}{\cancel{5} \text{ ml}}}{\underset{25}{\cancel{125} \text{ mg}}} = \frac{500 \text{ ml}}{25} = 20 \text{ ml}$$

R/P

$$125 \text{ mg} : 5 \text{ ml} :: 500 \text{ mg} : x \text{ ml}$$
$$125x = 5 \times 500$$
$$x = \frac{2,500}{125}$$
$$x = 20 \text{ ml}$$

22 Correct answer—**B**
Remember: 1 g = 1,000 mg

D/A

$$\underset{2}{\overset{1}{\cancel{500}}} \text{ mg} \times \frac{3 \text{ ml}}{1,\cancel{000} \text{ mg}} = \frac{3 \text{ ml}}{2} = 1.5 \text{ ml}$$

R/P

$$1,000 \text{ mg} : 3 \text{ ml} :: 500 \text{ mg} : x \text{ ml}$$
$$1,000x = 3 \times 500$$
$$x = \frac{1,500}{1,000}$$
$$x = 1.5 \text{ ml}$$

23 Correct answer—**A**

D/A

$$15 \text{ kg} \times \frac{0.01 \text{ mg}}{1 \text{ kg}} \times \frac{1 \text{ ml}}{0.3 \text{ mg}} = \frac{0.15 \text{ ml}}{0.3} = 0.5 \text{ ml}$$

R/P

Step 1: Calculate required milligrams.
$$1 \text{ kg} : 0.01 \text{ mg} :: 15 \text{ kg} : x \text{ mg}$$
$$x = 0.01 \times 15$$
$$x = 0.15 \text{ mg}$$

Step 2: Calculate required milliliters.
$$0.3 \text{ mg} : 1 \text{ ml} :: 0.15 \text{ mg} : x \text{ ml}$$
$$0.3x = 0.15$$
$$x = \frac{0.15}{0.3}$$
$$x = 0.5 \text{ ml}$$

24 Correct answer — **A**

D/A

$$\frac{30 \text{ mcgtt}}{1 \text{ min}} \times \frac{1 \text{ ml}}{\underset{1}{\cancel{60} \text{ mcgtt}}} \times \frac{\overset{1}{\cancel{60} \text{ min}}}{1 \text{ hr}} = 30 \text{ ml/hour}$$

R/P

Step 1: Change microdrops to milliliters.
$$60 \text{ mcgtt} : 1 \text{ ml} :: 30 \text{ mcgtt} : x \text{ ml}$$
$$60x = 30$$
$$x = \frac{30}{60}$$
$$x = 0.5 \text{ ml}$$

Step 2: Calculate milliliters per hour.
$$1 \text{ min} : 0.5 \text{ ml} :: 60 \text{ min} : x \text{ ml}$$
$$x = 0.5 \times 60$$
$$x = 30 \text{ ml/hour}$$

25 Correct answer — **C**

D/A

$$\overset{20}{\cancel{2,000}} \text{ ml} \times \frac{0.9 \text{ g}}{\underset{1}{\cancel{100} \text{ ml}}} = 18 \text{ g}$$

R/P

$$100 \text{ ml} : 0.9 \text{ g} :: 2,000 \text{ ml} : x \text{ g}$$
$$100x = 0.9 \times 2,000$$
$$x = \frac{1,800}{100}$$
$$x = 18 \text{ g}$$

26 Correct answer — **A**

D/A

$$200 \text{ mcg} \times \frac{1 \text{ mg}}{1,000 \text{ mcg}} \times \frac{1 \text{ tab}}{0.1 \text{ mg}} = \frac{200 \text{ tab}}{100} = 2 \text{ tablets}$$

R/P

Step 1: Change micrograms to milligrams.

$$1{,}000 \text{ mcg} : 1 \text{ mg} :: 200 \text{ mcg} : x \text{ mg}$$
$$1{,}000x = 200$$
$$x = \frac{200}{1{,}000}$$
$$x = 0.2 \text{ mg}$$

Step 2: Calculate required tablets.

$$0.1 \text{ mg} : 1 \text{ tab} :: 0.2 \text{ mg} : x \text{ tab}$$
$$0.1x = 0.2$$
$$x = \frac{0.2}{0.1}$$
$$x = 2 \text{ tablets}$$

---

27 Correct answer — C

D/A

$$65 \text{ kg} \times \frac{1.25 \text{ mg}}{1 \text{ kg}} \times \frac{\overset{1}{\cancel{10}} \text{ ml}}{\underset{5}{\cancel{50}} \text{ mg}} = \frac{81.25 \text{ ml}}{5} = 16.25 \text{ ml}$$

R/P

Step 1: Calculate required milligrams.

$$1 \text{ kg} : 1.25 \text{ mg} :: 65 \text{ kg} : x \text{ mg}$$
$$x = 1.25 \times 65$$
$$x = 81.25 \text{ mg}$$

Step 2: Calculate required milliliters.

$$50 \text{ mg} : 10 \text{ ml} :: 81.25 \text{ mg} : x \text{ ml}$$
$$50x = 10 \times 81.25$$
$$x = \frac{812.5}{50}$$
$$x = 16.25 \text{ ml}$$

---

28 Correct answer — C

D/A

$$\frac{250 \text{ ml}}{\underset{3}{\cancel{60}} \text{ min}} \times \frac{\overset{1}{\cancel{20}} \text{ gtt}}{1 \text{ ml}} = \frac{250 \text{ gtt}}{2 \text{ min}} = 83.3 \text{ or } 83 \text{ gtt/minute}$$

R/P

Step 1: Change milliliters to drops.
$$1 \text{ ml} : 20 \text{ gtt} :: 250 \text{ ml} : x \text{ gtt}$$
$$x = 20 \times 250$$
$$x = 5{,}000 \text{ gtt}$$

Step 2: Calculate the flow rate.
$$60 \text{ min} : 5{,}000 \text{ gtt} :: 1 \text{ min} : x \text{ gtt}$$
$$60x = 5{,}000$$
$$x = \frac{5{,}000}{60}$$
$$x = 83.3 \text{ or } 83 \text{ gtt/minute}$$

29 Correct answer—**D**

D/A

$$10 \ \cancel{\text{ml}} \times \frac{50 \ \cancel{\text{g}}}{\underset{1}{\cancel{100 \ \text{ml}}}} \times \frac{\overset{10}{\cancel{1{,}000 \text{ mg}}}}{1 \ \cancel{\text{g}}} = 5{,}000 \text{ mg}$$

R/P

Step 1: Calculate grams per 10 ml.
$$100 \text{ ml} : 50 \text{ g} :: 10 \text{ ml} : x \text{ g}$$
$$100x = 50 \times 10$$
$$x = \frac{500}{100}$$
$$x = 5 \text{ g}$$

Step 2: Change grams to milligrams.
$$1 \text{ g} : 1{,}000 \text{ mg} :: 5 \text{ g} : x \text{ mg}$$
$$x = 1{,}000 \times 5$$
$$x = 5{,}000 \text{ mg}$$

30 Correct answer—**C**

D/A

$$2.5\% = \frac{2.5}{100} = \frac{1}{40} \text{ or } 1{:}40$$

R/P

$$2.5 : 100 :: 1 : x$$
$$2.5x = 100$$
$$x = \frac{100}{2.5}$$
$$x = 40$$
Proportionate strength is 1:40

31 Correct answer—**B**

D/A

$$6 \text{ mg} \times \frac{\overset{1}{\cancel{10} \text{ ml}}}{\underset{5}{\cancel{50} \text{ mg}}} = \frac{6 \text{ ml}}{5} = 1.2 \text{ ml}$$

R/P

$$50 \text{ mg} : 10 \text{ ml} :: 6 \text{ mg} : x \text{ ml}$$
$$50x = 60$$
$$x = 60 \times 50$$
$$x = 1.2 \text{ ml}$$

32 Correct answer—**A**

D/A

$$0.03 \text{ g} \times \frac{1,000 \text{ mg}}{1 \text{ g}} \times \frac{1 \text{ tab}}{30 \text{ mg}} = \frac{30 \text{ tab}}{30} = 1 \text{ tablet}$$

R/P

$$1 \text{ g} : 1,000 \text{ mg} :: 0.03 \text{ g} : x \text{ mg}$$
$$x = 1,000 \times 0.03$$
$$x = 30 \text{ mg}$$

Because 30 mg = 1 tablet, give 1 tablet.

33 Correct answer—**C**

D/A

$$110 \text{ lb} \times \frac{1 \text{ kg}}{2.2 \text{ lb}} \times \frac{10 \text{ mg}}{1 \text{ kg}} = \frac{1,100 \text{ mg}}{2.2} = 500 \text{ mg}$$

R/P

Step 1: Change pounds to kilograms.
$$2.2 \text{ lb} : 1 \text{ kg} :: 110 \text{ lb} : x \text{ kg}$$
$$2.2x = 110$$
$$x = \frac{110}{2.2}$$
$$x = 50 \text{ kg}$$

Step 2: Calculate required milligrams.
$$1 \text{ kg} : 10 \text{ mg} :: 50 \text{ kg} : x \text{ mg}$$
$$x = 10 \times 50$$
$$x = 500 \text{ mg}$$

34 Correct answer—**B**

D/A

Remember: This is the standard formula.

$$\frac{°F - 32}{1.8} = °C$$

$$\frac{98.6 - 32}{1.8} = \frac{66.6}{1.8} = 37° \, C$$

35 Correct answer—**A**

D/A

$$0.05 \; \cancel{g} \times \frac{1,000 \; \cancel{mg}}{1 \; \cancel{g}} \times \frac{1 \; cap}{50 \; \cancel{mg}} = \frac{50 \; cap}{50} = 1 \; capsule$$

R/P

Step 1: Change grams to milligrams.

$$1 \; g : 1,000 \; mg :: 0.05 \; g : x \; mg$$
$$x = 1,000 \times 0.05$$
$$x = 50 \; mg$$

Step 2: Calculate required capsules.

Because 1 capsule = 50 mg, give 1 capsule.

36 Correct answer—**A**

D/A

$$40 \; \cancel{ml} \times \frac{\overset{1}{\cancel{50}} \; g}{\underset{2}{\cancel{100}} \; \cancel{ml}} = \frac{40 \; g}{2} = 20 \; g$$

R/P

$$100 \; ml : 50 \; g :: 40 \; ml : x \; g$$
$$100x = 50 \times 40$$
$$x = \frac{2,000}{100}$$
$$x = 20 \; g$$

37 Correct answer—**A**

D/A

$$\frac{1,000 \; \cancel{ml}}{16 \; \cancel{hr}} \times \frac{\overset{1}{\cancel{20}} \; gtt}{1 \; \cancel{ml}} \times \frac{1 \; \cancel{hr}}{\underset{3}{\cancel{60}} \; min} = \frac{1,000 \; gtt}{48} = 20.8 \; or \; 21 \; gtt/minute$$

R/P

Step 1: Change milliliters to drops.

$$1 \text{ ml} : 20 \text{ gtt} :: 1,000 \text{ ml} : x \text{ gtt}$$
$$x = 20 \times 1,000$$
$$x = 20,000 \text{ gtt}$$

Step 2: Change hours to minutes.

$$1 \text{ hr} : 60 \text{ min} :: 16 \text{ hr} : x \text{ min}$$
$$x = 60 \times 16$$
$$x = 960 \text{ minutes}$$

Step 3: Calculate the flow rate.

$$960 \text{ min} : 20,000 \text{ gtt} :: 1 \text{ min} : x \text{ gtt}$$
$$960x = 20,000$$
$$x = \frac{20,000}{960}$$
$$x = 20.8 \text{ or } 21 \text{ gtt/minute}$$

---

38 Correct answer — **A**

Remember: 1 g = 1,000 mg

D/A

$$70 \text{ kg} \times \frac{15 \text{ mg}}{1 \text{ kg}} \times \frac{2 \text{ ml}}{1,000 \text{ mg}} = \frac{2,100 \text{ ml}}{1,000} = 2.1 \text{ ml}$$

R/P

Step 1: Calculate required milligrams.

$$1 \text{ kg} : 15 \text{ mg} :: 70 \text{ kg} : x \text{ mg}$$
$$x = 15 \times 70$$
$$x = 1,050 \text{ mg}$$

Step 2: Calculate required milliliters.

$$1,000 \text{ mg} : 2 \text{ ml} :: 1,050 \text{ mg} : x \text{ ml}$$
$$1,000x = 2 \times 1,050$$
$$x = \frac{2,100}{1,000}$$
$$x = 2.1 \text{ ml}$$

---

39 Correct answer — **B**

D/A

$$0.5 \text{ g} \times \frac{15 \text{ ml}}{2 \text{ g}} = \frac{7.5 \text{ ml}}{2} = 3.75 \text{ ml}$$

R/P

$$2 \text{ g} : 15 \text{ ml} :: 0.5 \text{ g} : x \text{ ml}$$
$$2x = 15 \times 0.5$$
$$x = \frac{7.5}{2}$$
$$x = 3.75 \text{ ml}$$

40 Correct answer—C

D/A

$$\overset{34}{\cancel{340}} \ \cancel{\text{ml}} \times \frac{\overset{1}{\cancel{15}} \ \cancel{\text{gtt}}}{1 \ \cancel{\text{ml}}} \times \frac{1 \ \cancel{\text{min}}}{\underset{3}{\cancel{30}} \ \cancel{\text{gtt}}} \times \frac{1 \ \text{hr}}{\underset{4}{\cancel{60}} \ \cancel{\text{min}}} =$$

$$\frac{34 \text{ hr}}{12} = 2.83 \text{ hours or 2 hours, 50 minutes}$$

The I.V. infusion will end at 5:50 p.m.

R/P

Step 1: Change milliliters to drops.
$$1 \text{ ml} : 15 \text{ gtt} :: 340 \text{ ml} : x \text{ gtt}$$
$$x = 15 \times 340$$
$$x = 5{,}100 \text{ gtt}$$

Step 2: Calculate required minutes.
$$30 \text{ gtt} : 1 \text{ min} :: 5{,}100 \text{ gtt} : x \text{ min}$$
$$30x = 5{,}100$$
$$x = \frac{5{,}100}{30}$$
$$x = 170 \text{ minutes}$$

Step 3: Change minutes to hours.
$$60 \text{ min} : 1 \text{ hr} :: 170 \text{ min} : x \text{ hr}$$
$$60x = 170$$
$$x = \frac{170}{60}$$
$$x = 2.83 \text{ hours or 2 hours, 50 minutes}$$

The I.V. infusion will end at 5:50 p.m.

41 Correct answer—B

D/A

$$0.08 \ \cancel{\text{g}} \times \frac{1{,}000 \ \cancel{\text{mg}}}{1 \ \cancel{\text{g}}} \times \frac{1 \text{ tab}}{20 \ \cancel{\text{mg}}} = \frac{80 \text{ tab}}{20} = 4 \text{ tablets}$$

R/P

Step 1: Change grams to milligrams.

$$1 \text{ g} : 1{,}000 \text{ mg} :: 0.08 \text{ g} : x \text{ mg}$$
$$x = 1{,}000 \times 0.08$$
$$x = 80 \text{ mg}$$

Step 2: Calculate required tablets.

$$20 \text{ mg} : 1 \text{ tab} :: 80 \text{ mg} : x \text{ tab}$$
$$20x = 80$$
$$x = \frac{80}{20}$$
$$x = 4 \text{ tablets}$$

---

42 Correct answer — **C**

D/A

$$1.1 \ \cancel{m^2} \times \frac{0.075 \text{ mg}}{1 \ \cancel{m^2}} = 0.08 \text{ mg}$$

R/P

$$1 \text{ m}^2 : 0.075 \text{ mg} :: 1.1 \text{ m}^2 : x \text{ mg}$$
$$x = 0.075 \times 1.1$$
$$x = 0.08 \text{ mg}$$

---

43 Correct answer — **A**

D/A

$$2.75 \ \cancel{ml} \times \frac{2.5 \ \cancel{g}}{\overset{1}{\cancel{10 \ ml}}} \times \frac{\overset{100}{1{,}\cancel{000} \text{ mg}}}{1 \ \cancel{g}} = 687.5 \text{ or } 688 \text{ mg}$$

R/P

Step 1: Calculate required grams.

$$10 \text{ ml} : 2.5 \text{ g} :: 2.75 \text{ ml} : x \text{ g}$$
$$10x = 2.5 \times 2.75$$
$$x = \frac{6.875}{10}$$
$$x = 0.6875 \text{ g}$$

Step 2: Change grams to milligrams.

$$1 \text{ g} : 1{,}000 \text{ mg} :: 0.6875 \text{ g} : x \text{ mg}$$
$$x = 1{,}000 \times 0.6875$$
$$x = 687.5 \text{ or } 688 \text{ mg}$$

44 Correct answer — **D**

D/A

$$0.5 \text{ mg} \times \frac{1 \text{ tab}}{0.25 \text{ mg}} = \frac{0.5 \text{ tab}}{0.25} = 2 \text{ tablets}$$

R/P

$$0.25 \text{ mg} : 1 \text{ tab} :: 0.5 \text{ mg} : x \text{ tab}$$
$$0.25x = 0.5$$
$$x = \frac{0.5}{0.25}$$
$$x = 2 \text{ tablets}$$

45 Correct answer — **D**

D/A

$$0.004 \text{ g} \times \frac{1,000 \text{ mg}}{1 \text{ g}} \times \frac{1 \text{ tab}}{2 \text{ mg}} = \frac{4 \text{ tab}}{2} = 2 \text{ tablets}$$

R/P

$$1 \text{ g} : 1,000 \text{ mg} :: 0.004 \text{ g} : x \text{ mg}$$
$$x = 1,000 \times 0.004$$
$$x = 4 \text{ mg}$$

Because each tablet equals 2 mg, the patient must receive 2 tablets.

46 Correct answer — **D**

D/A

$$\frac{1 \text{ ml}}{1 \text{ min}} \times \frac{60 \text{ mcgtt}}{1 \text{ ml}} = 60 \text{ mcgtt/minute}$$

R/P

Step 1: Change milliliters to microdrops.
$$1 \text{ ml} : 60 \text{ mcgtt} :: 103 \text{ ml} : x \text{ mcgtt}$$
$$x = 60 \times 103$$
$$x = 6,180 \text{ mcgtt}$$

Step 2: Calculate the flow rate.
$$103 \text{ min} : 6,180 \text{ mcgtt} :: 1 \text{ min} : x \text{ mcgtt}$$
$$103x = 6,180$$
$$x = \frac{6,180}{103}$$
$$x = 60 \text{ mcgtt/minute}$$

47 Correct answer—**D**

D/A

$$0.75 \text{ g} \times \frac{1{,}000 \text{ mg}}{1 \text{ g}} \times \frac{1 \text{ ml}}{500 \text{ mg}} = \frac{750 \text{ ml}}{500} = 1.5 \text{ ml}$$

R/P

Step 1: Change grams to milligrams.

$$1 \text{ g} : 1{,}000 \text{ mg} :: 0.75 \text{ g} : x \text{ mg}$$
$$x = 1{,}000 \times 0.75$$
$$x = 750 \text{ mg}$$

Step 2: Calculate required milliliters.

$$500 \text{ mg} : 1 \text{ ml} :: 750 \text{ mg} : x \text{ ml}$$
$$500x = 750$$
$$x = \frac{750}{500}$$
$$x = 1.5 \text{ ml}$$

48 Correct answer—**C**

D/A

$$70 \text{ kg} \times \frac{0.5 \text{ mcg}}{\text{kg/min}} \times \frac{1 \text{ mg}}{\underset{2}{1{,}000 \text{ mcg}}} \times \frac{\overset{1}{500 \text{ ml}}}{\underset{5}{50 \text{ mg}}} \times \frac{\overset{6}{60 \text{ mcgtt}}}{1 \text{ ml}} =$$

$$\frac{210 \text{ mcgtt}}{10 \text{ min}} = 21 \text{ mcgtt/minute}$$

R/P

Step 1: Change milliliters to microdrops.

$$1 \text{ ml} : 60 \text{ mcgtt} :: 500 \text{ ml} : x \text{ mcgtt}$$
$$x = 60 \times 500$$
$$x = 30{,}000 \text{ mcgtt}$$

Step 2: Calculate required micrograms.

$$1 \text{ kg} : 0.5 \text{ mcg} :: 70 \text{ kg} : x \text{ mcg}$$
$$x = 0.5 \times 70$$
$$x = 35 \text{ mcg}$$

Step 3: Change micrograms to milligrams.

$$1{,}000 \text{ mcg} : 1 \text{ mg} :: 35 \text{ mcg} : x \text{ mg}$$
$$1{,}000x = 35$$
$$x = \frac{35}{1{,}000}$$
$$x = 0.035 \text{ mg}$$

Step 4: Calculate required minutes.

$$0.035 \text{ mg} : 1 \text{ min} :: 50 \text{ mg} : x \text{ min}$$
$$0.035x = 50$$
$$x = \frac{50}{0.035}$$
$$x = 1{,}428.5 \text{ minutes}$$

Step 5: Calculate the flow rate.

$$1{,}428.5 \text{ min} : 30{,}000 \text{ mcgtt} :: 1 \text{ min} : x \text{ mcgtt}$$
$$1{,}428.5x = 30{,}000$$
$$x = \frac{30{,}000}{1{,}428.5}$$
$$x = 21 \text{ mcgtt/minute}$$

49 Correct answer — D

D/A

Calculate the milliliters of drug to be added to the I.V. solution.

$$300 \text{ m\cancel{g}} \times \frac{1 \text{ ml}}{150 \text{ m\cancel{g}}} = \frac{300 \text{ ml}}{150} = 2 \text{ ml}$$

Calculate the flow rate for the total volume.

$$\frac{10 \text{ m\cancel{g}}}{1 \text{ min}} \times \frac{52 \text{ m\cancel{l}}}{\underset{5}{300} \text{ m\cancel{g}}} \times \frac{\overset{1}{\cancel{60}} \text{ mcgtt}}{1 \text{ m\cancel{l}}} = \frac{520 \text{ mcgtt}}{5 \text{ min}} = 104 \text{ mcgtt/minute}$$

R/P

Step 1: Calculate milliliters required.

$$150 \text{ mg} : 1 \text{ ml} :: 300 \text{ mg} : x \text{ ml}$$
$$150x = 300$$
$$x = \frac{300}{150}$$
$$x = 2 \text{ ml}$$

Step 2: Change milliliters to microdrops.

$$1 \text{ ml} : 60 \text{ mcgtt} :: 52 \text{ ml} : x \text{ mcgtt}$$
$$x = 60 \times 52$$
$$x = 3{,}120 \text{ mcgtt}$$

Step 3: Calculate required minutes.

$$10 \text{ mg} : 1 \text{ min} :: 300 \text{ mg} : x \text{ min}$$
$$10x = 300$$
$$x = \frac{300}{10}$$
$$x = 30 \text{ minutes}$$

Step 4: Calculate the flow rate.
$$30 \text{ min} : 3{,}120 \text{ mcgtt} :: 1 \text{ min} : x \text{ mcgtt}$$
$$30x = 3{,}120$$
$$x = \frac{3{,}120}{30}$$
$$x = 104 \text{ mcgtt/minute}$$

---

50 Correct answer—**B**

D/A

$$42 \cancel{\text{lb}} \times \frac{1 \cancel{\text{kg}}}{2.2 \cancel{\text{lb}}} \times \frac{\overset{1}{\cancel{5}} \cancel{\text{mg}}}{1 \cancel{\text{kg}}} \times \frac{1 \text{ tab}}{\underset{10}{\cancel{50}} \cancel{\text{mg}}} = \frac{42 \text{ tab}}{22} = 1.9 \text{ or 2 tablets}$$

R/P

Step 1: Change pounds to kilograms.
$$2.2 \text{ lb} : 1 \text{ kg} :: 42 \text{ lb} : x \text{ kg}$$
$$2.2x = 42$$
$$x = \frac{42}{2.2}$$
$$x = 19 \text{ kg}$$

Step 2: Calculate required milligrams.
$$1 \text{ kg} : 5 \text{ mg} :: 19 \text{ kg} : x \text{ mg}$$
$$x = 5 \times 19$$
$$x = 95 \text{ mg}$$

Step 3: Calculate required tablets.
$$50 \text{ mg} : 1 \text{ tab} :: 95 \text{ mg} : x \text{ tab}$$
$$50x = 95$$
$$x = \frac{95}{50}$$
$$x = 1.9 \text{ or 2 tablets}$$

---

51 Correct answer—**A**

D/A

$$\overset{2}{200} \cancel{\text{U}} \times \frac{1 \text{ ml}}{\underset{5}{\cancel{500}} \cancel{\text{U}}} = \frac{2 \text{ ml}}{5} = 0.4 \text{ ml}$$

R/P

$$500 \text{ U} : 1 \text{ ml} :: 200 \text{ U} : x \text{ ml}$$
$$500x = 200$$
$$x = \frac{200}{500}$$
$$x = 0.4 \text{ ml}$$

52 Correct answer — D

D/A

$$50 \text{ ml} \times \frac{1 \text{ min}}{1 \text{ ml}} = 50 \text{ minutes}$$

R/P

$$1 \text{ ml} : 1 \text{ min} :: 50 \text{ ml} : x \text{ min}$$
$$x = 1 \times 50$$
$$x = 50 \text{ minutes}$$

53 Correct answer — B

D/A

$$0.2 \text{ g} \times \frac{\overset{10}{1,000 \text{ mg}}}{1 \text{ g}} \times \frac{1 \text{ cap}}{\underset{1}{100 \text{ mg}}} = 2 \text{ capsules}$$

R/P

Step 1: Change grams to milligrams.
$$1 \text{ g} : 1,000 \text{ mg} :: 0.2 \text{ g} : x \text{ mg}$$
$$x = 1,000 \times 0.2$$
$$x = 200 \text{ mg}$$

Step 2: Calculate required capsules.
$$100 \text{ mg} : 1 \text{ cap} :: 200 \text{ mg} : x \text{ cap}$$
$$100x = 200$$
$$x = \frac{200}{100}$$
$$x = 2 \text{ capsules}$$

54 Correct answer — B

D/A

$$375 \text{ mg} \times \frac{1 \text{ tab}}{250 \text{ mg}} = \frac{375 \text{ tab}}{250} = 1.5 \text{ or } 1\frac{1}{2} \text{ tablets}$$

R/P

$$250 \text{ mg} : 1 \text{ tab} :: 375 \text{ mg} : x \text{ tab}$$
$$250x = 375$$
$$x = \frac{375}{250}$$
$$x = 1.5 \text{ or } 1\frac{1}{2} \text{ tablets}$$

55 Correct answer — C

D/A

$$1:4 = \frac{1}{4} = \frac{25}{100} = 25\%$$

$$\begin{array}{r} 25\% \\ -10\% \\ \hline 15\% \text{ difference} \end{array}$$

R/P

$$1 : 4 :: x : 100$$
$$4x = 100$$
$$x = \frac{100}{4}$$
$$x = 25\%$$

$$\begin{array}{r} 25\% \\ -10\% \\ \hline 15\% \text{ difference} \end{array}$$

56 Correct answer — C

D/A

$$24 \text{ hr} \times \frac{\overset{2}{\cancel{200} \text{ mg}}}{4 \text{ hr}} \times \frac{1 \text{ cap}}{\underset{1}{\cancel{100} \text{ mg}}} = \frac{48 \text{ cap}}{4} = 12 \text{ capsules}$$

R/P

$$4 \text{ hr} : 2 \text{ cap} :: 24 \text{ hr} : x \text{ cap}$$
$$4x = 24 \times 2$$
$$x = \frac{48}{4}$$
$$x = 12 \text{ capsules}$$

57 Correct answer — C

D/A

$$60 \text{ mg} \times \frac{1 \text{ ml}}{25 \text{ mg}} = \frac{60 \text{ ml}}{25} = 2.4 \text{ ml}$$

R/P

$$25 \text{ mg} : 1 \text{ ml} :: 60 \text{ mg} : x \text{ ml}$$
$$25x = 60$$
$$x = \frac{60}{25}$$
$$x = 2.4 \text{ ml}$$

58 Correct answer — **B**

D/A

$$1,20\!\!\!/0\!\!\!/,000 \;\cancel{U} \times \dfrac{1 \text{ ml}}{\dfrac{50\!\!\!/0\!\!\!/,000 \;\cancel{U}}{5}} \overset{12}{} = \dfrac{12 \text{ ml}}{5} = 2.4 \text{ ml}$$

R/P

$$500,000 \text{ U} : 1 \text{ ml} :: 1,200,000 \text{ U} : x \text{ ml}$$
$$500,000x = 1,200,000$$
$$x = \dfrac{1,200,000}{500,000}$$
$$x = 2.4 \text{ ml}$$

59 Correct answer — **D**

D/A

$$\dfrac{\overset{1}{50\!\!\!/0\!\!\!/ \;\cancel{mcg}}}{1 \text{ min}} \times \dfrac{1 \;\cancel{mg}}{\underset{2}{1,0\!\!\!/0\!\!\!/0\!\!\!/ \;\cancel{mcg}}} \times \dfrac{510 \;\cancel{ml}}{\underset{5}{10\!\!\!/0\!\!\!/ \;\cancel{mg}}} \times \dfrac{\overset{3}{6\!\!\!/0\!\!\!/ \text{ mcgtt}}}{1 \;\cancel{ml}} =$$

$$\dfrac{1,530 \text{ mcgtt}}{10 \text{ min}} = 153 \text{ mcgtt/minute}$$

R/P

Step 1: Change milliliters to microdrops.
$$1 \text{ ml} : 60 \text{ mcgtt} :: 510 \text{ ml} : x \text{ mcgtt}$$
$$x = 60 \times 510$$
$$x = 30,600 \text{ mcgtt}$$

Step 2: Calculate required milligrams.
$$1,000 \text{ mcg} : 1 \text{ mg} :: 50 \text{ mcg} : x \text{ mg}$$
$$1,000x = 500$$
$$x = \dfrac{500}{1,000}$$
$$x = 0.5 \text{ mg/minute}$$

Step 3: Calculate required minutes.
$$0.5 \text{ mg} : 1 \text{ min} :: 100 \text{ mg} : x \text{ min}$$
$$0.5x = 100$$
$$x = \dfrac{100}{0.5}$$
$$x = 200 \text{ minutes}$$

Step 4: Calculate the flow rate.

$$200 \text{ min} : 30{,}600 \text{ mcgtt} :: 1 \text{ min} : x \text{ mcgtt}$$
$$200x = 30{,}600$$
$$x = \frac{30{,}600}{200}$$
$$x = 153 \text{ mcgtt/minute}$$

60 Correct answer — C

D/A

$$40 \ \cancel{kg} \times \frac{25 \ \cancel{mg}}{1 \ \cancel{kg}} \times \frac{\overset{1}{\cancel{5}} \ ml}{\underset{10}{\cancel{50}} \ \cancel{mg}} = \frac{1{,}000 \ ml}{10} = 100 \ ml$$

R/P

Step 1: Calculate required milligrams.

$$1 \text{ kg} : 25 \text{ mg} :: 40 \text{ kg} : x \text{ mg}$$
$$x = 25 \times 40$$
$$x = 1{,}000 \text{ mg}$$

Step 2: Calculate required milliliters.

$$50 \text{ mg} : 5 \text{ ml} :: 1{,}000 \text{ mg} : x \text{ ml}$$
$$50x = 5 \times 1{,}000$$
$$x = \frac{5{,}000}{50}$$
$$x = 100 \text{ ml}$$

61 Correct answer — C

Remember: 1 g = 1,000 mg

D/A

$$\overset{100}{1{,}000} \ \cancel{mg} \times \frac{1 \ ml}{\underset{27}{\cancel{270}} \ \cancel{mg}} = \frac{100 \ ml}{27} = 3.7 \ ml$$

R/P

$$270 \text{ mg} : 1 \text{ ml} :: 1{,}000 \text{ mg} : x \text{ ml}$$
$$270x = 1{,}000$$
$$x = \frac{1{,}000}{270}$$
$$x = 3.7 \text{ ml}$$

62 Correct answer — **A**

Remember: A 25% solution is 25 g in 100 ml

D/A

$$2 \text{ vials} \times \frac{50 \text{ ml}}{1 \text{ vial}} \times \frac{\overset{1}{\cancel{25}} \text{ g}}{\underset{4}{\cancel{100}} \text{ ml}} = \frac{100 \text{ g}}{4} = 25 \text{ g}$$

R/P

$$50 \text{ ml} : 12.5 \text{ g} :: 100 \text{ ml} : x \text{ g}$$
$$50x = 12.5 \times 100$$
$$x = \frac{1,250}{50}$$
$$x = 25 \text{ g}$$

63 Correct answer — **A**

D/A

$$\overset{1}{\cancel{25}} \text{ mg} \times \frac{20 \text{ ml}}{\underset{40}{\cancel{1,000}} \text{ mg}} \times \frac{15 \text{ ℳ}}{1 \text{ ml}} = \frac{300 \text{ ℳ}}{40} = 7.5 \text{ ℳ}$$

R/P

Step 1: Calculate required milliliters.
$$1,000 \text{ mg} : 20 \text{ ml} :: 25 \text{ mg} : x \text{ ml}$$
$$1,000x = 20 \times 25$$
$$x = \frac{500}{1,000}$$
$$x = 0.5 \text{ ml}$$

Step 2: Change milliliters to minims.
$$1 \text{ ml} : 5 \text{ ℳ} :: 0.5 \text{ ml} : x \text{ ℳ}$$
$$x = 15 \times 0.5$$
$$x = 7.5 \text{ ℳ}$$

64 Correct answer — **D**

D/A

$$\cancel{400,000} \text{ U} \times \frac{1 \text{ ml}}{\cancel{200,000} \text{ U}} = \frac{4 \text{ ml}}{2} = 2 \text{ ml}$$

R/P

$$200,000 \text{ U} : 1 \text{ ml} :: 400,000 \text{ U} : x \text{ ml}$$
$$200,000x = 400,000$$
$$x = \frac{400,000}{200,000}$$
$$x = 2 \text{ ml}$$

65 Correct answer — **B**

D/A

$$75 \; \cancel{mg} \times \frac{1 \; tab}{37.5 \; \cancel{mg}} = \frac{75 \; tab}{37.5} = 2 \; tablets$$

R/P

$$37.5 \; mg : 1 \; tab :: 75 \; mg : x \; tab$$
$$37.5x = 75$$
$$x = \frac{75}{37.5}$$
$$x = 2 \; tablets$$

66 Correct answer — **A**

D/A

$$\frac{100 \; \cancel{ml}}{\underset{1}{\cancel{30}} \; min} \times \frac{\overset{2}{\cancel{60}} \; mcgtt}{1 \; \cancel{ml}} = 200 \; mcgtt/minute$$

R/P

Step 1: Change milliliters to microdrops.
$$1 \; ml : 60 \; mcgtt :: 100 \; ml : x \; mcgtt$$
$$x = 60 \times 100$$
$$x = 6,000 \; mcgtt$$

Step 2: Calculate the flow rate.
$$30 \; min : 6,000 \; mcgtt :: 1 \; min : x \; mcgtt$$
$$30x = 6,000$$
$$x = \frac{6,000}{30}$$
$$x = 200 \; mcgtt/minute$$

67 Correct answer — **D**

D/A

$$70 \; \cancel{kg} \times \frac{\overset{1}{\cancel{10}} \; \cancel{mg}}{1 \; \cancel{kg}} \times \frac{1 \; ml}{\underset{40}{\cancel{400}} \; \cancel{mg}} = \frac{70 \; ml}{40} = 1.75 \; ml$$

R/P

Step 1: Calculate required milligrams.
$$1 \; kg : 10 \; mg :: 70 \; kg : x \; kg$$
$$x = 10 \times 70$$
$$x = 700 \; mg$$

Step 2: Calculate required milliliters.

$$400 \text{ mg} : 1 \text{ ml} :: 700 \text{ mg} : x \text{ mg}$$
$$400x = 700$$
$$x = \frac{700}{400}$$
$$x = 1.75 \text{ ml}$$

68 Correct answer — B

D/A

$$\overset{1}{\cancel{20}} \cancel{U} \times \frac{1 \text{ ml}}{\underset{5}{\cancel{100}} \cancel{U}} = \frac{1 \text{ ml}}{5} = 0.2 \text{ ml}$$

R/P

$$100 \text{ U} : 1 \text{ ml} :: 20 \text{ U} : x \text{ ml}$$
$$100x = 20$$
$$x = \frac{20}{100}$$
$$x = 0.2 \text{ ml}$$

69 Correct answer — C

D/A

$$\frac{\overset{10}{\cancel{100}} \cancel{ml}}{\underset{3}{\cancel{30}} \text{ min}} \times \frac{20 \text{ gtt}}{1 \cancel{ml}} = \frac{200 \text{ gtt}}{3 \text{ min}} = 66.6 \text{ or } 67 \text{ gtt/minute}$$

R/P

Step 1: Change milliliters to drops.

$$1 \text{ ml} : 20 \text{ gtt} :: 100 \text{ ml} : x \text{ gtt}$$
$$x = 20 \times 100$$
$$x = 2,000 \text{ gtt}$$

Step 2: Calculate the flow rate.

$$30 \text{ min} : 2,000 \text{ gtt} :: 1 \text{ min} : x \text{ gtt}$$
$$30x = 2,000$$
$$x = \frac{2,000}{30}$$
$$x = 66.6 \text{ or } 67 \text{ gtt/minute}$$

70 Correct answer — B

D/A

$$0.25 \cancel{g} \times \frac{\overset{2}{\cancel{1,000}} \cancel{mg}}{1 \cancel{g}} \times \frac{1 \text{ ml}}{\underset{1}{\cancel{500}} \cancel{mg}} = 0.5 \text{ ml}$$

R/P

Step 1: Change grams to milligrams.

$$1 \text{ g} : 1{,}000 \text{ mg} :: 0.25 \text{ g} : x \text{ mg}$$
$$x = 1{,}000 \times 0.25$$
$$x = 250 \text{ mg}$$

Step 2: Calculate required milliliters.

$$500 \text{ mg} : 1 \text{ ml} :: 250 \text{ mg} : x \text{ ml}$$
$$500x = 250$$
$$x = \frac{250}{500}$$
$$x = 0.5 \text{ ml}$$

---

71 Correct answer — **C**

D/A

$$66 \; \cancel{\text{kg}} \times \frac{0.3 \; \cancel{\text{mg}}}{1 \; \cancel{\text{kg}}} \times \frac{1 \text{ ml}}{10 \; \cancel{\text{mg}}} = \frac{19.8 \text{ ml}}{10} \text{ or } 1.98 \text{ or } 2 \text{ ml}$$

R/P

Step 1: Calculate required milligrams.

$$1 \text{ kg} : 0.3 \text{ mg} :: 66 \text{ kg} : x \text{ mg}$$
$$x = 0.3 \times 66$$
$$x = 19.8 \text{ mg}$$

Step 2: Calculate required milliliters.

$$10 \text{ mg} : 1 \text{ ml} :: 19.8 \text{ mg} : x \text{ ml}$$
$$10x = 19.8$$
$$x = \frac{19.8}{10}$$
$$x = 1.98 \text{ or } 2 \text{ ml}$$

---

72 Correct answer — **B**

D/A

$$0.2 \; \cancel{\text{g}} \times \frac{1{,}000 \; \cancel{\text{mg}}}{1 \; \cancel{\text{g}}} \times \frac{1 \text{ tab}}{100 \; \cancel{\text{mg}}} = \frac{200 \text{ tab}}{100} = 2 \text{ tablets}$$

R/P

Step 1: Change grams to milligrams.

$$1 \text{ g} : 1{,}000 \text{ mg} :: 0.2 \text{ g} : x \text{ mg}$$
$$x = 1{,}000 \times 0.2$$
$$x = 200 \text{ mg}$$

Step 2: Calculate required tablets.

$$100 \text{ mg} : 1 \text{ tab} :: 200 \text{ mg} : x \text{ tab}$$
$$100x = 200$$
$$x = \frac{200}{100}$$
$$x = 2 \text{ tablets}$$

73 Correct answer — D

D/A

$$15 \, \cancel{g} \times \frac{1 \text{ tsp}}{3.75 \, \cancel{g}} = \frac{15 \text{ tsp}}{3.75} = 4 \text{ tsp}$$

R/P

$$3.75 \text{ g} : 1 \text{ tsp} :: 15 \text{ g} : x \text{ tsp}$$
$$3.75x = 15$$
$$x = \frac{15}{3.75}$$
$$x = 4 \text{ tsp}$$

74 Correct answer — D

D/A

$$625 \, \cancel{ml} \times \frac{\overset{1}{\cancel{60}} \text{ mcgtt}}{1 \, \cancel{ml}} \times \frac{1 \, \cancel{min}}{100 \text{ mcgtt}} \times \frac{1 \text{ hr}}{\underset{1}{\cancel{60}} \, \cancel{min}} =$$

$$\frac{625 \text{ hr}}{100} = 6.25 \text{ hours or 6 hours, 15 minutes}$$

R/P

Step 1: Change milliliters to microdrops.

$$1 \text{ ml} : 60 \text{ mcgtt} :: 625 \text{ ml} : x \text{ mcgtt}$$
$$x = 60 \times 625$$
$$x = 37,500 \text{ mcgtt}$$

Step 2: Calculate required minutes.

$$100 \text{ mcgtt} : 1 \text{ min} :: 37,500 \text{ mcgtt} : x \text{ min}$$
$$100x = 37,500$$
$$x = \frac{37,500}{100}$$
$$x = 375 \text{ minutes}$$

Step 3: Change minutes to hours.

$$60 \text{ min} : 1 \text{ hr} :: 375 \text{ min} : x \text{ hr}$$
$$60x = 375$$
$$x = \frac{375}{60}$$
$$x = 6.25 \text{ hours or 6 hours, 15 minutes}$$

75

Correct answer — **A**

Remember: 1 gr = 60 mg

D/A

$$\frac{1 \cancel{mg}}{10 \text{ min}} \times \frac{1,000 \cancel{ml}}{\underset{1}{\cancel{60} \cancel{mg}}} \times \frac{\overset{1}{\cancel{60}} \text{ mcgtt}}{1 \cancel{ml}} = 100 \text{ mcgtt/minute}$$

R/P

Step 1: Change milliliters to microdrops.

$$1 \text{ ml} : 60 \text{ mcgtt} :: 1,000 \text{ ml} : x \text{ mcgtt}$$
$$x = 60 \times 1,000$$
$$x = 60,000 \text{ mcgtt}$$

Step 2: Calculate required minutes.

$$1 \text{ mg} : 10 \text{ min} :: 60 \text{ mg} : x \text{ min}$$
$$x = 10 \times 60$$
$$x = 600 \text{ minutes}$$

Step 3: Calculate the flow rate.

$$600 \text{ min} : 60,000 \text{ mcgtt} :: 1 \text{ min} : x \text{ mcgtt}$$
$$600x = 60,000$$
$$x = \frac{60,000}{600}$$
$$x = 100 \text{ mcgtt/minute}$$

76

Correct answer — **B**

D/A

$$0.52 \cancel{m^2} \times \frac{5 \text{ mg}}{1 \cancel{m^2}} = 2.6 \text{ mg}$$

R/P

$$1 \text{ m}^2 : 5 \text{ mg} :: 0.52 \text{ m}^2 : x \text{ mg}$$
$$x = 5 \times 0.52$$
$$x = 2.6 \text{ mg}$$

77 Correct answer — C

Remember: 2.5 cm = 1″

D/A

$$22 \ \cancel{mg} \times \frac{1''}{15 \ \cancel{mg}} = \frac{22''}{15} = 1.46 \text{ or } 1\frac{1}{2}''$$

R/P

$$15 \text{ mg} : 1'' :: 22 \text{ mg} : x''$$
$$15x = 22$$
$$x = \frac{22}{15}$$
$$x = 1.46 \text{ or } 1\frac{1}{2}''$$

78 Correct answer — B

D/A

$$\frac{150 \ \overset{}{\cancel{ml}}}{\underset{3}{\cancel{90} \text{ min}}} \times \frac{\overset{2}{\cancel{60} \text{ mcgtt}}}{1 \ \cancel{ml}} = \frac{300 \text{ mcgtt}}{3 \text{ min}} = 100 \text{ mcgtt/minute}$$

R/P

Step 1: Change milliliters to microdrops.

$$1 \text{ ml} : 60 \text{ mcgtt} :: 150 \text{ ml} : x \text{ mcgtt}$$
$$x = 60 \times 150$$
$$x = 9,000 \text{ mcgtt}$$

Step 2: Calculate the flow rate.

$$90 \text{ min} : 9,000 \text{ mcgtt} :: 1 \text{ min} : x \text{ mcgtt}$$
$$90x = 9,000$$
$$x = \frac{9,000}{90}$$
$$x = 100 \text{ mcgtt/minute}$$

79 Correct answer — C

D/A

$$\frac{13 \ \overset{}{\cancel{U}}}{\underset{1}{\cancel{60} \text{ min}}} \times \frac{\overset{4}{1,\cancel{000} \ \cancel{ml}}}{\underset{1}{\cancel{250} \ \cancel{U}}} \times \frac{\overset{1}{\cancel{60} \text{ mcgtt}}}{1 \ \cancel{ml}} = 52 \text{ mcgtt/minute}$$

R/P

Step 1: Change milliliters to microdrops.

$$1 \text{ ml} : 60 \text{ mcgtt} :: 1{,}000 \text{ ml} : x \text{ mcgtt}$$
$$x = 60 \times 1{,}000$$
$$x = 60{,}000 \text{ mcgtt}$$

Step 2: Calculate required minutes.

$$13 \text{ U} : 60 \text{ min} :: 250 \text{ U} : x \text{ min}$$
$$13x = 60 \times 250$$
$$x = \frac{15{,}000}{13}$$
$$x = 1{,}153.8 \text{ minutes}$$

Step 3: Calculate the flow rate.

$$1{,}153.8 \text{ min} : 60{,}000 \text{ mcgtt} :: 1 \text{ min} : x \text{ mcgtt}$$
$$1{,}153.8x = 60{,}000$$
$$x = \frac{60{,}000}{1{,}153.8}$$
$$x = 52 \text{ mcgtt/minute}$$

80 Correct answer — **D**

D/A

$$20 \ \cancel{\text{kg}} \times \frac{0.25 \text{ ml}}{1 \ \cancel{\text{kg}}} = 5 \text{ ml}$$

R/P

$$1 \text{ kg} : 0.25 \text{ ml} :: 20 \text{ kg} : x \text{ ml}$$
$$x = 0.25 \times 20$$
$$x = 5 \text{ ml}$$

81 Correct answer — **A**

D/A

$$\frac{100 \ \cancel{\text{ml}}}{\overset{}{\underset{4}{\cancel{60}} \text{ min}}} \times \frac{\overset{1}{\cancel{15}} \text{ gtt}}{1 \ \cancel{\text{ml}}} = \frac{100 \text{ gtt}}{4 \text{ min}} = 25 \text{ gtt/minute}$$

R/P

Step 1: Change milliliters to drops.

$$1 \text{ ml} : 15 \text{ gtt} :: 100 \text{ ml} : x \text{ gtt}$$
$$x = 15 \times 100$$
$$x = 1{,}500 \text{ gtt}$$

Step 2: Calculate the flow rate.
$$60 \text{ min} : 1{,}500 \text{ gtt} :: 1 \text{ min} : x \text{ gtt}$$
$$60x = 1{,}500$$
$$60x = 1{,}500$$
$$x = \frac{1{,}500}{60}$$
$$x = 25 \text{ gtt/minute}$$

82 Correct answer — **B**

D/A

$$0.7 \ \cancel{m^2} \times \frac{75 \text{ mg}}{\cancel{m^2}} = 52.5 \text{ mg}$$

R/P

$$1 \text{ m}^2 : 75 \text{ mg} :: 0.7 \text{ m}^2 : x \text{ mg}$$
$$x = 75 \times 0.7$$
$$x = 52.5 \text{ mg}$$

83 Correct answer — **D**

D/A

$$\frac{5 \ \cancel{gr}}{2} \times \frac{\overset{6}{\cancel{60} \ \cancel{mg}}}{1 \ \cancel{gr}} \times \frac{1 \text{ supp}}{\underset{10}{\cancel{100} \ \cancel{mg}}} = \frac{30 \text{ supp}}{20} = 1.5 \text{ or } 1\tfrac{1}{2} \text{ suppositories}$$

Because suppositories should not be split, call the pharmacy to supply the correct strength.

R/P

Step 1: Change grains to milligrams.
$$1 \text{ gr} : 60 \text{ mg} :: 2.5 \text{ gr} : x \text{ mg}$$
$$x = 60 \times 2.5$$
$$x = 150 \text{ mg}$$

Step 2: Calculate required suppositories.
$$100 \text{ mg} : 1 \text{ supp} :: 150 \text{ mg} : x \text{ supp}$$
$$100x = 150 \text{ mg}$$
$$x = \frac{150}{100}$$
$$x = 1.5 \text{ or } 1\tfrac{1}{2} \text{ suppositories}$$

Because suppositories should not be split, call the pharmacy to supply the correct strength.

84 Correct answer — **A**

D/A

$$2 \, \cancel{g} \times \frac{\overset{2}{\cancel{100} \text{ ml}}}{\underset{1}{\cancel{50} \, \cancel{g}}} = 4 \text{ ml}$$

R/P

$$50 \text{ g} : 100 \text{ ml} :: 2 \text{ g} : x \text{ ml}$$
$$50x = 100 \times 2$$
$$x = \frac{200}{50}$$
$$x = 4 \text{ ml}$$

85 Correct answer — **D**

D/A

$$\overset{1}{\cancel{500} \text{ mg}} \times \frac{1 \, \cancel{g}}{\underset{2}{\cancel{1,000} \text{ mg}}} \times \frac{\overset{2}{\cancel{100} \text{ ml}}}{\underset{1}{\cancel{50} \, \cancel{g}}} = \frac{2 \text{ ml}}{2} = 1 \text{ ml}$$

R/P

Step 1: Change milligrams to grams.
$$1,000 \text{ g} : 1 \text{ g} :: 500 \text{ mg} : x \text{ g}$$
$$1,000x = 500$$
$$x = \frac{500}{1,000}$$
$$x = 0.5 \text{ g}$$

Step 2: Calculate required milliliters.
$$50 \text{ g} : 100 \text{ ml} :: 0.5 \text{ g} : x \text{ ml}$$
$$50x = 100 \times 0.5$$
$$x = \frac{50}{50}$$
$$x = 1 \text{ ml}$$

86 Correct answer — **A**

D/A

$$52.3 \, \cancel{kg} \times \frac{0.3 \, \cancel{U}}{\cancel{kg}/\text{min}} \times \frac{\overset{1}{\cancel{1,000} \text{ ml}}}{\underset{20}{\cancel{20,000} \, \cancel{U}}} \times \frac{20 \text{ gtt}}{1 \, \cancel{ml}} =$$

$$\frac{313.8 \text{ gtt}}{20 \text{ min}} = 15.6 \text{ or } 16 \text{ gtt/minute}$$

R/P

Step 1: Change milliliters to drops.

$$1 \text{ ml} : 20 \text{ gtt} :: 1{,}000 \text{ ml} : x \text{ gtt}$$
$$x = 20 \times 1{,}000$$
$$x = 20{,}000 \text{ gtt}$$

Step 2: Calculate required units.

$$1 \text{ kg} : 0.3 \text{ U} :: 52.3 \text{ kg} : x \text{ U}$$
$$x = 0.3 \times 52.3$$
$$x = 15.69 \text{ U}$$

Step 3: Calculate required minutes.

$$15.69 \text{ U} : 1 \text{ min} :: 20{,}000 \text{ U} : x \text{ min}$$
$$15.69 \, x = 20{,}000$$
$$x = \frac{20{,}000}{15.69}$$
$$x = 1{,}274.6 \text{ minutes}$$

Step 4: Calculate the flow rate.

$$1{,}274.6 \text{ min} : 20{,}000 \text{ gtt} :: 1 \text{ min} : x \text{ gtt}$$
$$1{,}274.6x = 20{,}000$$
$$x = \frac{20{,}000}{1{,}274.6}$$
$$x = 15.6 \text{ or } 16 \text{ gtt/minute}$$

87 Correct answer — **C**

D/A

$$75 \ \cancel{kg} \times \frac{0.01 \ \cancel{mcg}}{\cancel{kg}/min} \times \frac{\overset{2}{\cancel{50} \ \cancel{ml}}}{\underset{1}{\cancel{25} \ \cancel{mcg}}} \times \frac{60 \ mcgtt}{1 \ \cancel{ml}} = 90 \ mcgtt/minute$$

R/P

Step 1: Change milliliters to microdrops.

$$1 \text{ ml} : 60 \text{ mcgtt} :: 50 \text{ ml} : x \text{ mcgtt}$$
$$x = 60 \times 50$$
$$x = 3{,}000 \text{ mcgtt}$$

Step 2: Calculate required micrograms.

$$1 \text{ kg} : 0.01 \text{ mcg} :: 75 \text{ kg} : x \text{ mcg}$$
$$x = 0.01 \times 75$$
$$x = 0.75 \text{ mcg}$$

Step 3: Calculate required minutes.

$$0.75 \text{ mcg} : 1 \text{ min} :: 25 \text{ mcg} : x \text{ min}$$
$$0.75x = 25$$
$$x = \frac{25}{0.75}$$
$$x = 33.3 \text{ minutes}$$

Step 4: Calculate the flow rate.

$$33.3 \text{ min} : 3{,}000 \text{ mcgtt} :: 1 \text{ min} : x \text{ mcgtt}$$
$$33.3x = 3{,}000$$
$$x = \frac{3{,}000}{33.3}$$
$$x = 90 \text{ mcgtt/minute}$$

88 Correct answer — **D**

D/A

$$66 \; \cancel{kg} \times \frac{0.02 \; \cancel{mg}}{1 \; \cancel{kg}/min} \times \frac{\overset{2}{\cancel{1{,}000} \; \cancel{ml}}}{\underset{1}{\cancel{500} \; \cancel{mg}}} \times \frac{20 \text{ gtt}}{1 \; \cancel{ml}} = 52.8 \text{ or } 53 \text{ gtt/minute}$$

R/P

Step 1: Change milliliters to drops.

$$1 \text{ ml} : 20 \text{ gtt} :: 1{,}000 \text{ ml} : x \text{ gtt}$$
$$x = 20 \times 1{,}000$$
$$x = 20{,}000 \text{ gtt}$$

Step 2: Calculate required milligrams.

$$1 \text{ kg} : 0.02 \text{ mg} :: 66 \text{ kg} : x \text{ mg}$$
$$x = 0.02 \times 66$$
$$x = 1.32 \text{ mg}$$

Step 3: Calculate required minutes.

$$1.32 \text{ mg} : 1 \text{ min} :: 500 \text{ mg} : x \text{ min}$$
$$1.32x = 500$$
$$x = \frac{500}{1.32}$$
$$x = 378.7 \text{ minutes}$$

Step 4: Calculate the flow rate.

$$378.7 \text{ min} : 20{,}000 \text{ gtt} :: 1 \text{ min} : x \text{ gtt}$$
$$378.7x = 20{,}000$$
$$x = \frac{20{,}000}{378.7}$$
$$x = 52.8 \text{ or } 53 \text{ gtt/minute}$$

89 Correct answer — **A**

D/A

$$40.9 \; \cancel{kg} \times \frac{0.015 \; \cancel{mg}}{\cancel{kg}/min} \times \frac{\overset{20}{\cancel{1{,}000} \; \cancel{ml}}}{\underset{3}{\cancel{150} \; \cancel{mg}}} \times \frac{15 \text{ gtt}}{1 \; \cancel{ml}} =$$

$$\frac{184.05 \text{ gtt}}{3 \text{ min}} = 61.3 \text{ or } 61 \text{ gtt/minute}$$

R/P

Step 1: Change milliliters to drops.

$$1 \text{ ml} : 15 \text{ gtt} :: 1{,}000 \text{ ml} : x \text{ gtt}$$
$$x = 15 \times 1{,}000$$
$$x = 15{,}000 \text{ gtt}$$

Step 2: Calculate required milligrams.

$$1 \text{ kg} : 0.015 \text{ mg} :: 40.9 \text{ kg} : x \text{ mg}$$
$$x = 0.015 \times 40.9$$
$$x = 0.6135 \text{ mg}$$

Step 3: Calculate required minutes.

$$0.6135 \text{ mg} : 1 \text{ min} :: 150 \text{ mg} : x \text{ min}$$
$$0.6135x = 150$$
$$x = \frac{150}{0.6135}$$
$$x = 244.4 \text{ minutes}$$

Step 4: Calculate the flow rate.

$$244.4 \text{ min} : 15{,}000 \text{ gtt} :: 1 \text{ min} : x \text{ gtt}$$
$$244.4x = 15{,}000$$
$$x = \frac{15{,}000}{244.4}$$
$$x = 61.3 \text{ or } 61 \text{ gtt/minute}$$

90 Correct answer — A

D/A

$$54.5 \ \cancel{\text{kg}} \times \frac{0.05 \ \cancel{\text{mg}}}{\cancel{\text{kg}}/\text{min}} \times \frac{\overset{4}{\cancel{200}} \ \cancel{\text{ml}}}{\underset{3}{\cancel{150}} \ \cancel{\text{mg}}} \times \frac{10 \text{ gtt}}{1 \ \cancel{\text{ml}}} =$$

$$\frac{109 \text{ gtt}}{3 \text{ min}} = 36.3 \text{ or } 36 \text{ gtt/minute}$$

R/P

Step 1: Change milliliters to drops.

$$1 \text{ ml} : 10 \text{ gtt} :: 200 \text{ ml} : x \text{ gtt}$$
$$x = 10 \times 200$$
$$x = 2{,}000 \text{ gtt}$$

Step 2: Calculate required milligrams.

$$1 \text{ kg} : 0.05 \text{ mg} :: 54.5 \text{ kg} : x \text{ mg}$$
$$x = 0.05 \times 54.5$$
$$x = 2.725 \text{ mg}$$

Step 3: Calculate required minutes.

$$2.725 \text{ mg} : 1 \text{ min} :: 150 \text{ mg} : x \text{ min}$$
$$2.725x = 150$$
$$x = \frac{150}{2.725}$$
$$x = 55 \text{ minutes}$$

Step 4: Calculate the flow rate.

$$55 \text{ min} : 2,000 \text{ gtt} :: 1 \text{ min} : x \text{ gtt}$$
$$55x = 2,000$$
$$x = \frac{2,000}{55}$$
$$x = 36.3 \text{ or } 36 \text{ gtt/minute}$$

91 Correct answer — **D**

D/A

$$195 \text{ lb} \times \frac{1 \text{ kg}}{2.2 \text{ lb}} \times \frac{0.5 \text{ mcg}}{\text{kg/min}} \times \frac{1 \text{ mg}}{1,000 \text{ mcg}} \times \frac{\overset{1}{1,000} \text{ ml}}{\underset{5}{50} \text{ mg}} \times \frac{\overset{2}{20} \text{ gtt}}{1 \text{ ml}} =$$

$$\frac{195 \text{ gtt}}{11 \text{ min}} = 17.7 \text{ or } 18 \text{ gtt/minute}$$

R/P

Step 1: Change milliliters to drops.

$$1 \text{ ml} : 20 \text{ gtt} :: 1,000 \text{ ml} : x \text{ gtt}$$
$$x = 20 \times 1,000$$
$$x = 20,000 \text{ gtt}$$

Step 2: Change pounds to kilograms.

$$2.2 \text{ lb} : 1 \text{ kg} :: 195 \text{ lb} : x \text{ kg}$$
$$2.2x = 195$$
$$x = \frac{195}{2.2}$$
$$x = 88.63 \text{ kg}$$

Step 3: Calculate required micrograms.

$$1 \text{ kg} : 0.5 \text{ mcg} :: 88.63 \text{ kg} : x \text{ mcg}$$
$$x = 0.5 \times 88.63$$
$$x = 44.3 \text{ mcg}$$

Step 4: Change micrograms to milligrams.

$$1,000 \text{ mcg} : 1 \text{ mg} :: 44.3 \text{ mcg} : x \text{ mg}$$
$$1,000x = 44.3$$
$$x = \frac{44.3}{1,000}$$
$$x = 0.0443 \text{ mg/minute}$$

Step 5: Calculate required minutes.
$$0.0443 \text{ mg} : 1 \text{ min} :: 50 \text{ mg} : x \text{ min}$$
$$0.0443x = 50$$
$$x = \frac{50}{0.0443}$$
$$x = 1{,}128.6 \text{ minutes}$$

Step 6: Calculate the flow rate.
$$1{,}128.6 \text{ min} : 20{,}000 \text{ gtt} :: 1 \text{ min} : x \text{ gtt}$$
$$1{,}128.6x = 20{,}000$$
$$x = \frac{20{,}000}{1{,}128.6}$$
$$x = 17.7 \text{ or } 18 \text{ gtt/minute}$$

92 Correct answer — **B**

D/A

$$116 \text{ lb} \times \frac{1 \text{ kg}}{2.2 \text{ lb}} \times \frac{5.6 \text{ mg}}{\underset{3}{\text{kg}/30 \text{ min}}} \times \frac{\overset{1}{100 \text{ ml}}}{\underset{3}{300 \text{ mg}}} \times \frac{\overset{1}{10 \text{ gtt}}}{1 \text{ ml}} =$$

$$\frac{649.6 \text{ gtt}}{19.8 \text{ min}} = 32.8 \text{ or } 33 \text{ gtt/minute}$$

R/P

Step 1: Change milliliters to drops.
$$1 \text{ ml} : 10 \text{ gtt} :: 100 \text{ ml} : x \text{ gtt}$$
$$x = 10 \times 100$$
$$x = 1{,}000 \text{ gtt}$$

Step 2: Change pounds to kilograms.
$$2.2 \text{ lb} : 1 \text{ kg} :: 116 \text{ lb} : x \text{ kg}$$
$$2.2x = 116$$
$$x = \frac{116}{2.2}$$
$$x = 52.7 \text{ kg}$$

Step 3: Calculate required milligrams.
$$1 \text{ kg} : 5.6 \text{ mg} :: 52.7 \text{ kg} : x \text{ mg}$$
$$x = 5.6 \times 52.7$$
$$x = 295.1 \text{ mg}$$

Step 4: Calculate required minutes.
$$295.1 \text{ mg} : 30 \text{ min} :: 300 \text{ mg} : x \text{ min}$$
$$295.1x = 30 \times 300$$
$$x = \frac{9{,}000}{295.1}$$
$$x = 30.49 \text{ minutes}$$

Step 5: Calculate the flow rate.

$$30.49 \text{ min} : 1,000 \text{ gtt} :: 1 \text{ min} : x \text{ gtt}$$
$$30.49x = 1,000$$
$$x = \frac{1,000}{30.49}$$
$$x = 32.79 \text{ or } 33 \text{ gtt/minute}$$

93 Correct answer—**B**

D/A

$$154 \cancel{lb} \times \frac{1 \cancel{kg}}{2.2 \cancel{lb}} \times \frac{50 \cancel{U}}{\underset{6}{\cancel{kg}/\cancel{60} \text{ min}}} \times \frac{\overset{1}{\cancel{500} \cancel{ml}}}{\underset{10}{5,000 \cancel{U}}} \times \frac{\overset{1}{\cancel{10} \text{ gtt}}}{1 \cancel{ml}} =$$

$$\frac{7,700 \text{ gtt}}{132 \text{ min}} = 58.3 \text{ or } 58 \text{ gtt/minute}$$

R/P

Step 1: Change milliliters to drops.

$$1 \text{ ml} : 10 \text{ gtt} :: 500 \text{ ml} : x \text{ gtt}$$
$$x = 10 \times 500$$
$$x = 5,000 \text{ gtt}$$

Step 2: Change pounds to kilograms.

$$2.2 \text{ lb} : 1 \text{ kg} :: 154 \text{ lb} : x \text{ kg}$$
$$2.2x = 154$$
$$x = \frac{154}{2.2}$$
$$x = 70 \text{ kg}$$

Step 3: Calculate required units.

$$1 \text{ kg} : 50 \text{ U} :: 70 \text{ kg} : x \text{ U}$$
$$x = 50 \times 70$$
$$x = 3,500 \text{ U}$$

Step 4: Calculate required minutes.

$$3,500 \text{ U} : 60 \text{ min} :: 5,000 \text{ U} : x \text{ min}$$
$$3,500x = 60 \times 5,000$$
$$x = \frac{300,000}{3,500}$$
$$x = 85.7 \text{ minutes}$$

Step 5: Calculate the flow rate.

$$85.7 \text{ min} : 5,000 \text{ gtt} :: 1 \text{ min} : x \text{ gtt}$$
$$85.7x = 5,000$$
$$x = \frac{5,000}{85.7}$$
$$x = 58.3 \text{ or } 58 \text{ gtt/minute}$$

94 Correct answer—**A**

D/A

$$142 \text{ lb} \times \frac{1 \text{ kg}}{2.2 \text{ lb}} \times \frac{0.03 \text{ mcg}}{\text{kg/min}} \times \frac{\overset{1}{500} \text{ ml}}{\underset{4}{2,000} \text{ mcg}} \times \frac{60 \text{ mcgtt}}{1 \text{ ml}} =$$

$$\frac{255.6 \text{ mcgtt}}{8.8 \text{ min}} = 28.9 \text{ or } 29 \text{ mcgtt/minute}$$

R/P

Step 1: Change milliliters to microdrops.

$$1 \text{ ml} : 60 \text{ mcgtt} :: 500 \text{ ml} : x \text{ mcgtt}$$
$$x = 60 \times 500$$
$$x = 30,000 \text{ gtt}$$

Step 2: Change pounds to kilograms.

$$2.2 \text{ lb} : 1 \text{ kg} :: 142 \text{ lb} : x \text{ kg}$$
$$2.2x = 142$$
$$x = \frac{142}{2.2}$$
$$x = 64.54 \text{ kg}$$

Step 3: Calculate required micrograms.

$$1 \text{ kg} : 0.03 \text{ mcg} :: 64.54 \text{ kg} : x \text{ mcg}$$
$$x = 0.03 \times 64.54$$
$$x = 1.93 \text{ mcg}$$

Step 4: Change micrograms to milligrams.

$$1,000 \text{ mcg} : 1 \text{ mg} :: 1.93 \text{ mcg} : x \text{ mg}$$
$$1,000x = 1.93$$
$$x = \frac{1.93}{1,000}$$
$$x = 0.00193 \text{ mg/minute}$$

Step 5: Calculate required minutes.

$$0.00193 \text{ mg} : 1 \text{ min} :: 2 \text{ mg} : x \text{ min}$$
$$0.00193x = 2$$
$$x = \frac{2}{0.00193}$$
$$x = 1,036.2 \text{ minutes}$$

Step 6: Calculate the flow rate.

$$1036.2 \text{ min} : 30,000 \text{ gtt} :: 1 \text{ min} : x \text{ gtt}$$
$$1036.2x = 30,000$$
$$x = \frac{30,000}{1,036.2}$$
$$x = 28.9 \text{ or } 29 \text{ mcgtt/minute}$$

95
Correct answer—**A**

D/A

$$125 \text{ lb} \times \frac{1 \text{ kg}}{2.2 \text{ lb}} \times \frac{0.004 \text{ mg}}{\text{kg/min}} \times \frac{\overset{2}{1,000} \text{ ml}}{\underset{1}{500} \text{ mg}} \times \frac{20 \text{ gtt}}{1 \text{ ml}} =$$

$$\frac{20 \text{ gtt}}{2.2 \text{ min}} = 9.09 \text{ or } 9 \text{ gtt/minute}$$

R/P

Step 1: Change milliliters to drops.

$$1 \text{ ml} : 20 \text{ gtt} :: 1,000 \text{ ml} : x \text{ gtt}$$
$$x = 20 \times 1,000$$
$$x = 20,000 \text{ gtt}$$

Step 2: Change pounds to kilograms.

$$2.2 \text{ lb} : 1 \text{ kg} :: 125 \text{ lb} : x \text{ kg}$$
$$2.2x = 125$$
$$x = \frac{125}{2.2}$$
$$x = 56.8 \text{ kg}$$

Step 3: Calculate required milligrams.

$$1 \text{ kg} : 0.004 \text{ mg} :: 56.8 \text{ kg} : x \text{ mg}$$
$$x = 0.004 \times 56.8$$
$$x = 0.227 \text{ mg}$$

Step 4: Calculate required minutes.

$$0.227 \text{ mg} : 1 \text{ min} :: 500 \text{ mg} : x \text{ min}$$
$$0.227x = 500$$
$$x = \frac{500}{0.227}$$
$$x = 2,202.6 \text{ minutes}$$

Step 5: Calculate the flow rate.

$$2,202.6 \text{ min} : 20,000 \text{ gtt} :: 1 \text{ min} : x \text{ gtt}$$
$$2,202.6x = 20,000$$
$$x = \frac{20,000}{2,202.6}$$
$$x = 9.1 \text{ or } 9 \text{ gtt/minute}$$

96 Correct answer — **B**

D/A

$$64 \,\cancel{lb} \times \frac{1 \,\cancel{kg}}{2.2 \,\cancel{lb}} \times \frac{0.3 \,\cancel{mg}}{\cancel{kg}/30 \text{ min}} \times \frac{\overset{4}{\cancel{120}} \,\cancel{ml}}{\underset{1}{\cancel{60}} \,\cancel{mg}} \times \frac{\overset{1}{\cancel{60}} \text{ mcgtt}}{1 \,\cancel{ml}} =$$

$$\frac{76.8 \text{ mcgtt}}{2.2 \text{ min}} = 34.8 \text{ or } 35 \text{ mcgtt/minute}$$

R/P

Step 1: Change milliliters to microdrops.

$$1 \text{ ml} : 60 \text{ mcgtt} :: 120 \text{ ml} : x \text{ mcgtt}$$
$$x = 60 \times 120$$
$$x = 7,200 \text{ gtt}$$

Step 2: Change pounds to kilograms.

$$2.2 \text{ lb} : 1 \text{ kg} :: 64 \text{ lb} : x \text{ kg}$$
$$2.2x = 64$$
$$x = \frac{64}{2.2}$$
$$x = 29 \text{ kg}$$

Step 3: Calculate required milligrams.

$$1 \text{ kg} : 0.3 \text{ mg} :: 29 \text{ kg} : x \text{ mg}$$
$$x = 0.3 \times 29$$
$$x = 8.7 \text{ mg}$$

Step 4: Calculate required minutes.

$$8.7 \text{ mg} : 30 \text{ min} :: 60 \text{ mg} : x \text{ min}$$
$$8.7x = 30 \times 60$$
$$x = \frac{1,800}{8.7}$$
$$x = 206.8 \text{ minutes}$$

Step 5: Calculate the flow rate.

$$206.8 \text{ min} : 7,200 \text{ mcgtt} :: 1 \text{ min} : x \text{ mcgtt}$$
$$206.8x = 7,200$$
$$x = \frac{7,200}{206.8}$$
$$x = 34.8 \text{ or } 35 \text{ mcgtt/minute}$$

97

Correct answer—**B**

D/A

$$110 \not{lb} \times \frac{1 \not{kg}}{2.2 \not{lb}} \times \frac{0.8 \not{mcg}}{\not{kg}/min} \times \frac{\overset{1}{\cancel{500}} \not{ml}}{\underset{10}{\cancel{5,000}} \not{mcg}} \times \frac{10 \text{ gtt}}{1 \not{ml}} =$$

$$\frac{880 \text{ gtt}}{22 \text{ min}} = 40 \text{ gtt/minute}$$

R/P

Step 1: Change milliliters to drops.

$$1 \text{ ml} : 10 \text{ gtt} :: 500 \text{ ml} : x \text{ gtt}$$
$$x = 10 \times 500$$
$$x = 5,000 \text{ gtt}$$

Step 2: Change pounds to kilograms.

$$2.2 \text{ lb} : 1 \text{ kg} :: 100 \text{ lb} : x \text{ kg}$$
$$2.2x = 110$$
$$x = \frac{110}{2.2}$$
$$x = 50 \text{ kg}$$

Step 3: Calculate required micrograms.

$$1 \text{ kg} : 0.8 \text{ mcg} :: 50 \text{ kg} : x \text{ mcg}$$
$$x = 0.8 \times 50$$
$$x = 40 \text{ mcg}$$

Step 4: Change micrograms to milligrams.

$$1,000 \text{ mcg} : 1 \text{ mg} :: 40 \text{ mcg} : x \text{ mg}$$
$$1,000x = 40$$
$$x = \frac{40}{1,000}$$
$$x = 0.04 \text{ mg}$$

Step 5: Calculate required minutes.

$$0.04 \text{ mg} : 1 \text{ min} :: 5 \text{ mg} : x \text{ min}$$
$$0.04x = 5$$
$$x = \frac{5}{0.04}$$
$$x = 125 \text{ minutes}$$

Step 6: Calculate the flow rate.

$$125 \text{ min} : 5,000 \text{ gtt} :: 1 \text{ min} : x \text{ gtt}$$
$$125x = 5,000$$
$$x = \frac{5,000}{125}$$
$$x = 40 \text{ gtt/minute}$$

98 Correct answer — C

D/A

$$138 \ \text{lb} \times \frac{1 \ \text{kg}}{2.2 \ \text{lb}} \times \frac{6.5 \ \text{mcg}}{\text{kg/min}} \times \frac{1 \ \text{mg}}{\overset{1}{1{,}000 \ \text{mcg}}} \times \frac{\overset{1}{1{,}000 \ \text{ml}}}{\underset{25}{500 \ \text{mg}}} \times$$

$$\frac{\overset{3}{60} \ \text{mcgtt}}{1 \ \text{ml}} = \frac{2{,}691 \ \text{mcgtt}}{55 \ \text{min}} = 48.9 \ \text{or} \ 49 \ \text{mcgtt/minute}$$

R/P

Step 1: Change milliliters to microdrops.

$$1 \ \text{ml} : 60 \ \text{mcgtt} :: 1{,}000 \ \text{ml} : x \ \text{mcgtt}$$
$$x = 60 \times 1{,}000$$
$$x = 60{,}000 \ \text{mcgtt}$$

Step 2: Change pounds to kilograms.

$$2.2 \ \text{lb} : 1 \ \text{kg} :: 138 \ \text{lb} : x \ \text{kg}$$
$$2.2x = 138$$
$$x = \frac{138}{2.2}$$
$$x = 62.72 \ \text{kg}$$

Step 3: Calculate required micrograms.

$$1 \ \text{kg} : 6.5 \ \text{mcg} :: 62.72 \ \text{kg} : x \ \text{mcg}$$
$$x = 6.5 \times 62.72$$
$$x = 407.7 \ \text{mcg}$$

Step 4: Change micrograms to milligrams.

$$1{,}000 \ \text{mcg} : 1 \ \text{mg} :: 407.7 \ \text{mcg} : x \ \text{mg}$$
$$1{,}000x = 407.7$$
$$x = \frac{407.7}{1{,}000}$$
$$x = 0.4077 \ \text{mg}$$

Step 5: Calculate required minutes.

$$0.4077 \ \text{mg} : 1 \ \text{min} :: 500 \ \text{mg} : x \ \text{min}$$
$$0.4077x = 500$$
$$x = \frac{500}{0.4077}$$
$$x = 1{,}226.3 \ \text{minutes}$$

Step 6: Calculate the flow rate.

$$1{,}226.3 \ \text{min} : 60{,}000 \ \text{mcgtt} :: 1 \ \text{min} : x \ \text{mcgtt}$$
$$1{,}226.3x = 60{,}000$$
$$x = \frac{60{,}000}{1{,}226.3}$$
$$x = 48.9 \ \text{or} \ 49 \ \text{mcgtt/minute}$$

99 Correct answer—**A**

D/A

$$72 \text{ kg} \times \frac{3 \text{ mcg}}{\text{kg/min}} \times \frac{1 \text{ mg}}{\underset{200}{1{,}000 \text{ mcg}}} \times \frac{\overset{101}{5\cancel{0}5} \text{ ml}}{\underset{20}{4\cancel{0}0 \text{ mg}}} \times \frac{\overset{3}{60 \text{ min}}}{1 \text{ hr}} =$$

$$\frac{65{,}448 \text{ ml}}{4{,}000 \text{ hr}} = 16.3 \text{ ml/hour}$$

R/P

Step 1: Calculate required micrograms.

$$1 \text{ kg} : 3 \text{ mcg} :: 72 \text{ kg} : x \text{ mcg}$$
$$x = 3 \times 72$$
$$x = 216 \text{ mcg}$$

Step 2: Change micrograms to milligrams.

$$1{,}000 \text{ mcg} : 1 \text{ mg} :: 216 \text{ mcg} : x \text{ mg}$$
$$1{,}000x = 216$$
$$x = \frac{216}{1{,}000}$$
$$x = 0.216 \text{ mg}$$

Step 3: Calculate required milliliters.

$$400 \text{ mg} : 505 \text{ ml} :: 0.216 \text{ mg} : x \text{ ml}$$
$$400x = 505 \times 0.216$$
$$x = \frac{109.08}{400}$$
$$x = 0.27 \text{ ml}$$

Step 4: Calculate the flow rate.

$$1 \text{ min} : 0.27 \text{ ml} :: 60 \text{ min} : x \text{ ml}$$
$$x = 0.27 \times 60$$
$$x = 16.3 \text{ ml/hour}$$

100 Correct answer — **A**

D/A

$$72 \; \cancel{kg} \times \frac{0.002 \; \cancel{mg}}{\cancel{kg}/\cancel{min}} \times \frac{505 \; ml}{\underset{20}{\cancel{400} \; \cancel{mg}}} \times \frac{\overset{3}{\cancel{60} \; \cancel{min}}}{1 \; hr} =$$

$$\frac{218.1 \; ml}{20 \; hr} = 10.9 \; ml/hour$$

R/P

Step 1: Calculate required milligrams.

$$1 \; kg : 0.002 \; mg :: 72 \; kg : x \; mg$$
$$x = 0.002 \times 72$$
$$x = 0.144 \; mg$$

Step 2: Calculate required milliliters.

$$400 \; mg : 505 \; ml :: 0.144 \; mg : x \; ml$$
$$400x = 505 \times 0.144$$
$$x = \frac{72.72}{400}$$
$$x = 0.181 \; ml$$

Step 3: Calculate milliliters per hour.

$$1 \; min : 0.181 \; ml :: 60 \; min : x \; ml$$
$$x = 0.181 \times 60$$
$$x = 10.9 \; ml/hour$$

Appendix: Common Abbreviations in Drug Therapy

The following abbreviations commonly appear in physicians' orders and, depending on institutional policy, may be used in transcribing medication orders and documenting drug administration.

b.i.d.	twice a day	**m**	meter
c	cup	**mcg**	microgram
C	centigrade, Celsius	**mEq**	milliequivalent
cap	capsule	**mg**	milligram
cc	cubic centimeter	**mgtt**	microdrop or minidrop
cm	centimeter	**ml**	milliliter
d	day	**mm**	millimeter
D₅W	dextrose 5% in water	**M_x or ℳ**	minim
f℥	fluidram	**N.P.O.**	nothing by mouth
f℥	fluidounce	**oz or ℥**	ounce
F	Fahrenheit	**P.O.**	by mouth
ft or '	foot	**pt**	pint
g	gram	**q**	every
gr	grain	**q.i.d.**	four times a day
gtt	drop	**qt**	quart
h or hr	hour	**S.C.**	subcutaneous
I.M.	intramuscular	**ss**	one-half
in or "	inch	**supp**	suppository
I.V.	intravenous	**Tbs, tbsp**	tablespoon
IVPB	intravenous "piggyback"	**tsp**	teaspoon
kg	kilogram	**tab**	tablet
L	liter	**t.i.d.**	three times a day
lb	pound	**x**	times, multiply

Selected References

American Hospital Formulary Service, Bethesda, Md.: American Society of Hospital Pharmacists, 1990.

Baer, C., and Williams, B. *Clinical Pharmacology and Nursing.* Springhouse, Pa.: Springhouse Corp., 1988.

Physicians' Desk Reference, 45th ed. Oradell, N.J.: Medical Economics Co., 1991.

Skidmore, L. *Mosby's Nursing Drug Reference, 1991.* St. Louis: C.V. Mosby Co., 1990.

Springhouse Drug Reference. Springhouse, Pa.: Springhouse Corp., 1989.